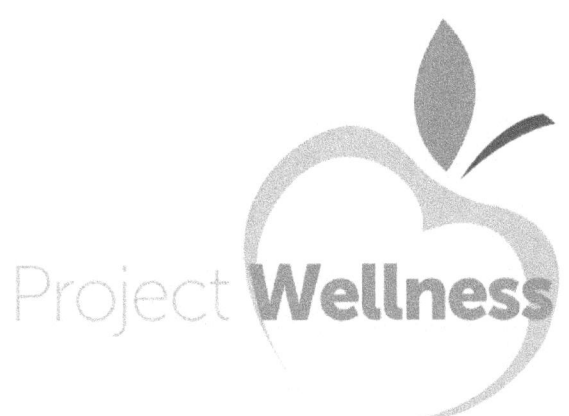

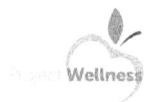

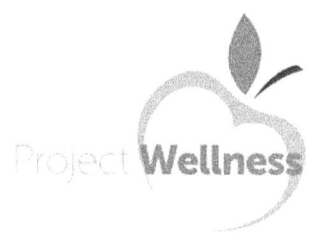

# DEDICATION

To all those who have taught me about wellness and how to ultimately
achieve it and sustain it.

To the patients who have shared many difficult journeys with me, and
to the mentors and coaches who have helped me understand the ways
of the human body and how to crack the code of wellness and
sustainable weight loss.

To my husband, Bryan, for believing in me, for teaching me that
anything is possible with positive thinking, and for loving me
unconditionally.

To my son, who always makes me laugh and teaches me to see God as
doing things "for me" and not "to me."

To my family, for their sacrifices while I made this trek, and for
supporting me in every way.

To God, who created me perfectly to share this message with the world
and works with me constantly to grow into what He created me to be.

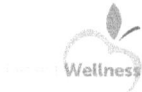

For Information about permissions to reproduce selections from this book or to purchase copies for educational, business or sales promotional use, contact:

Project Wellness
5212 Village Parkway
Rogers, AR 72758
479-657-6888

First Edition

Printed in the USA
ISBN-13: 978-1502967879

ISBN-10: 1502967871

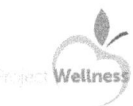

# TABLE OF CONTENTS

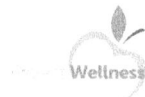

Wellness

## Hi and welcome!

If you are reading this, you are either "sick and tired of being sick and tired," or you are staring at a family history of all sorts of unwanted things and asking yourself, "How can I prevent what's in my DNA from activating in a way that may affect my quality of life?"

How do you want your life to look a year from today? I once heard this analogy for life. Imagine holding eighty pennies in your hand. Not that many, right? You could easily hold eighty pennies. Feel the cold hard metal and the faint smell of copper and dirt as they slip through your fingers. Well, if you are lucky, you get eighty pennies.

That's eighty years of your life. Eighty summers, eighty springs, eighty birthdays, eighty Christmases. Eighty years is just not that many. If you are reaching your midlife, how many pennies do you have now? Forty, maybe fifty. If you are fifty like me that's only thirty pennies left. How do I want to spend them?

Quality of life is everything. My mom is in assisted living and has Alzheimer's. I was there one evening coloring her hair and it took about two hours. As I was leaving, she said, "When are you going to come back and color my hair?"

That upset me terribly. I barely made it home before bursting into tears. I called my brother sobbing, and he listened to my rant.

"I am upset about mom," I told him, almost out of breath. "But I'm conflicted because we saw her mom die of Alzheimer's, and it was so horrible. Now mom, and then I start wondering… When me? Every time I lose my keys or forget something, I panic a little. When me?"

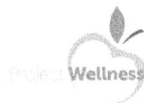

"Oh, Tammy," he said gently. "I see your choices you make every day. Every bite of food you put in your mouth. You exercise every day. You take care of your hormones and your mind. That won't be you. You understand that, right?"

And in that moment, I knew he was right. That my choices would trump my genetics. And that has become my "why." Taking care of myself is important to avoid those terrible manifestations of memory loss. With a family history of both Alzheimer's and cancer, I don't want my young son to have to deal with what I have seen in my family members.

And so every day I make those choices to eat healthy, to exercise, to take care of my hormones and my mind.

You can do that, too, and it's never too late to start. I have some patients ask me, "Am I too old?" I tell them I have seen miracle after miracle. I have seen eighty-year-old diabetics cure their diabetes and neuropathy. I have seen the elderly regain their sex lives, feel young again, and play with their grandchildren. There are even tons of elderly folks that start bodybuilding in their seventies and eighties.

You make the choice. You make the choice with all your little choices, and they all add up. When will you start making more beneficial choices than detrimental ones? That is when you decide what you want your quality of life to look like.

When I was in high school, I hurt all the time. I told my parents, and they told me it was just growing pains. I had no idea why I hurt so deep and ached in my joints and muscles.

When I was in college, I checked out the school infirmary and asked the doctor to run some tests. Not just any tests because I had done my homework. I looked up almost three thousand dollars worth of lab tests from autoimmune to inflammation markers to try to find out why I hurt so much.

I waited three long weeks and finally got the call from the nurse at the clinic. "Your labs are normal." She said cheerily on the phone.

"What?!" I screamed inside. "How could they be normal?" There had to be something wrong. I felt horrible and hurt from head to toe. Even my little toe hurt!

My husband tried to console me, and in a moment of truth, he told me, "You know, honey, you eat absolutely horrible! Maybe you should change your diet a little. At least take some vitamins."

I realized he was right. All I ever ate was junk. I was raised that way. My parents worked a lot and they just did the best they could. Captain Crunch for breakfast, mac 'n' cheese for lunch, McDonalds for dinner.

I had an ah-ha moment and immediately went to the health food store, bought some vitamins and started eating more of a Paleo low sugar diet. I felt amazing within two weeks. That was the first time I understood the impact of "You are what you eat!"

Today I help people realize that wherever they are, they can feel better and prevent disease. Of course we will all die of something, but when and with what quality is totally dependent on your choices.

My goal is to help everyone start feeling better, so here is your quick start. Make these changes over the next 3 weeks and you will feel stronger, more alive, more vibrant, and more powerful than you have in years.

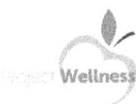

## Quick Start

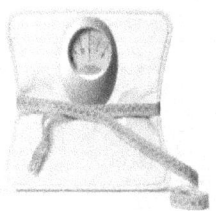

# 3 Week/3 Steps Quick Start

Welcome to the Project Wellness Program! Based on the 5 pillars of a well-balanced life—Hormones, Nutrition, Fitness, Stress, and Detox—we want you to get a jump start on feeling better!

**The first step is to define your goals.**

My first 3 goals are:

_____

_____

_____

Why?

_____

_____

_____

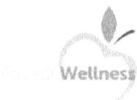

Starting your hormone balance depends on going to the source of all imbalance and is based on 3 easy steps: 1) What you eat, 2) Nutrient/Vitamin/Mineral Supplementation, and 3) Fitness.

Drink at least 64 oz. of water a day. Drink a full 8 oz. on rising in the morning.

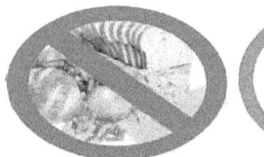 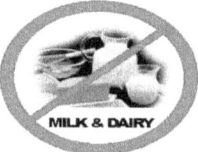

**Empowering hormone balance foods:**
Target Hormones: Insulin (reduce simple sugars), Leptin (5 small meals a day) and reducing Cortisol (avoid gluten and dairy).

Start with a protein shake in the morning, and plan meals and snacks. Eat 5 small meals a day to increase Leptin sensitivity, the hormone that maximizes fat burning.
Avoid the two most common inflammatory foods: Gluten and Dairy.

Foods you should eat include lean protein (think chicken breasts, eggs, and wild-caught fish); vegetables and most fruit; chia seeds, flaxseeds, and most nuts; olive oil and some other unsaturated oils and fats, like coconut oil; and whole grains like buckwheat, brown rice, and quinoa.

Avoid or minimize caffeine, alcohol, fried foods, processed meat, peanuts, saturated or hydrogenated fat, dairy, artificial sweeteners, sodas, and simple carbs.

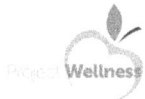

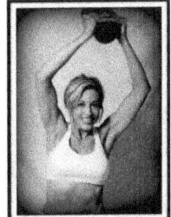**Metabolic Support Supplements are very important:**
Omega-3 fatty acids
Magnesium
Methyl-B12
Methyl-Folate
Iodine

**Fitness:**
Time commitment, 11 minutes a day

Traditionally, it is believed that in order to burn fat, classic cardio is the ideal form of exercise. The problem is with that type of exercise, you are in a slow fat burning mode only during the time of exercise. With metabolic conditioning, you stimulate the hormones that increase metabolism and elicit the body to be in fat burning mode for up to 24-48 hours, post-exercise. This is known as the after-burn effect. The most effective fat burning exercise is High Intensity Interval Training. This exercise system elicits a very unique hormonal response in the body, and ultimately, it is your hormones that influence your metabolism. This type of exercise is called "metabolic conditioning." Metabolic conditioning is characterized by short bursts of high intensity exercise. Therefore, in just minutes a day, you can build muscle and burn fat like never before. Eleven minutes a day is all it takes to get in the shape of your life. Project Wellness High Intensity program is a

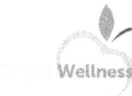

get-fit-for-life program.  We incorporate all the essential characteristics of fitness, including power, strength, endurance, balance, coordination, flexibility, speed, and agility.

(First make sure that you are healthy enough to exercise by getting a physical medical examination from your doctor.)

    1. Put on some really fast music and get a timer.

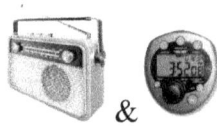
&

    2.  Stretch lightly for 30 seconds
    3.  Do the following exercises for 11 minutes in intervals.

20 seconds run in place as HARD as you can
20 seconds rest

20 seconds punch in the air as hard as you can
20 seconds rest

20 seconds get up and down from a chair as fast as you can
20 seconds rest

Repeat circuit x 5 then a 1 minute cool down/stretch
Or do a combination of the following exercises in 20 minute cycles as above.
Mix and match to avoid getting bored.

Crunches
Jumping Jacks
Weighted or resistance exercises.
Journal what exercises you do each day to keep track and introduce variety.

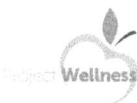

# Introduction

### What is Project Wellness?

Project Wellness is just that, a PROJECT. A project to develop a way of thinking that challenges you to make a commitment to consider your health and wellness a priority by taking advantage of education, enlightenment, and empowering ideals that we have to offer. Our program will give every BODY the best chance of transformation of reaching your health, wellness, weight loss, and fitness goals.

Typically, other programs address only one of the following physical areas: nutrition, food, or exercise. We believe for a life-sustaining transformation to occur, three components must be addressed that include physical, emotional, and spiritual (mind, body, and spirit):

1. Physical: includes medical, food/nutrition, and exercise
2. Emotional: includes an awareness of how emotions can play a big part of overall wellness, metabolic, and weight loss strategies to address this critical area. The great divide between bliss and stress is important to understand to find balance in your life and focus on finding the bliss more than the stressful reactions.
3. Spiritual: offers an awareness or perspective regarding the importance of engaging God or a power greater than self to find a deeper understanding of our significance.

We refer to these components as the three-legged stool, without one you fall down—it takes all three.

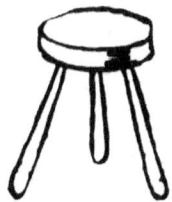

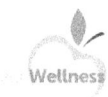
And we combine these in the physical framework of what we call "The 5 Pillars of Health," which address:

1. Nutrition
2. Detoxing the system
3. Fitness
4. Hormone Balance
5. Stress

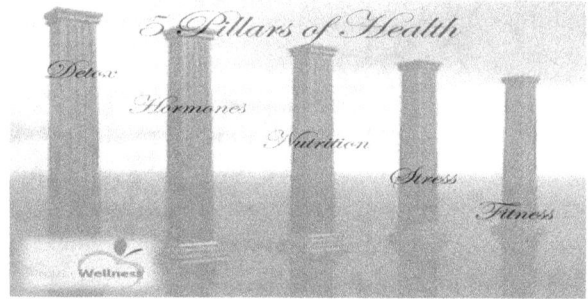

**What are the benefits of Project Wellness?**

There is no other program that we are aware of that addresses the physical (Nutrition, detox, fitness, hormone balance and stress), the emotional, and the spiritual components of wellness.

The benefits of Project Wellness are many. The program begins with the physical (metabolic) and emotional/psychological aspects that are vital to sustainable wellness and weight loss. It is essential to treat all patients as individuals. The blood never lies and it is important to obtain some lab levels to find out your metabolic status, nutritional status, food sensitivities, and hormone status. Finding this out can explain current hormone levels and imbalances that have been possibly preventing you from weight loss or causing weight gain in the past. Nine out of ten of our patients usually have some type of hormone imbalances and food sensitivities.

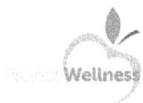

Over the past eight years, I have seen patients lose hundreds of pounds. People have transformed before my very eyes. Marriages have been healed from the ravages of hormonally imbalanced women AND men. I have been given a gift to be able to help people through this journey. I have sought out every aspect of metabolic realignment I could, and this is the simplest presentation I have come up with.

The principles are really quite simple, although the nuances can be tricky. You will need a physician on your side willing to go the distance and pay attention to the details.

The goal of this book is to teach you the basic principles and empower you to explore them in the context of your own health. It is not meant to be a replacement for medical care; rather, a tool you can use to enlighten your own physician about subjects we are not taught in medical school. My main priority is you experience the three "E"s to the fullest: educate, enlighten, and empower.

Education is the first step. Explore new territories. Never stop learning. With education, you can be taught, but never really enlightened. This is the next step. To truly understand what you have educated yourself about, then you are truly empowered to start your journey. Healing, like life, is a journey, not a destination. I hope you enjoy the ride!

I truly practice what I preach because the bottom line is: Project Wellness is completely "doable." There is nothing complicated or difficult about the program.

The hardest part is making the commitment to change and then BELIEVE you can do it!

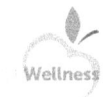

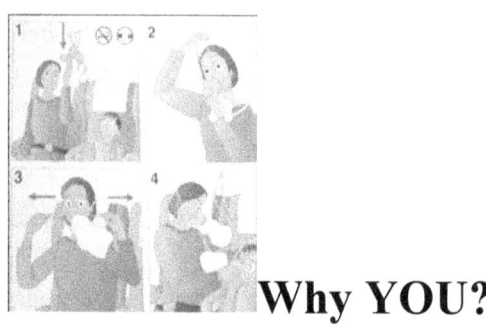

# Why YOU?

Consider this...

When there is a sudden change in cabin pressure during an airline flight and the oxygen mask drops down, what are you supposed to do?

You put the mask on yourself, FIRST!

Why? Because if you don't take care of yourself first, you can't take care of or help anyone else.
If you lose consciousness, you can't put the mask on your child or dependent loved one.

You have to put yourself first.

This may go against everything you think or believe, but if you are not healthy, you lose your effectiveness with your children, your spouse, your work, and even yourself.

Project Wellness is about taking care of yourself so that you can take control and make a difference in the lives of everyone around you.

When you make positive changes in your life, your children will learn from your healthy choices.

Start today by choosing to be healthy and take control of your life.

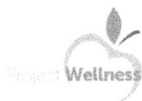

ARE YOU READY?

So many of us invest years of our lives learning how to be something: a doctor, artist, teacher, nurse, business executive, electrician, or any other career that you wanted to pursue.

But we spend almost no time learning HOW to be the best something we can!

How much time do we actually spend developing our inner being or searching out how to be fabulous? Feeling our best is essential for success, productivity, creativity, innovation, relationship success, health, and almost everything else in life! We usually wait for a life crisis or tragedy that forces us to look at what is really important. But is this really the best approach for change and growth?

The best approach is a proactive approach to hardwire our brains with focus, awareness, repetition, and celebration.

Isn't it time to be a fabulous celebration of your changed life!

Not to mention sharing it with others on a similar journey!

Practicing the daily exercises can change the way your brain is wired.

Imagine how different you, your life, your brain—and more importantly—YOUR HEART will be when you have completed all 5 Pillars of Project Wellness.

Who is the program for?

Anyone who wants to take charge of your health and wellness.

If you want to be your ideal body composition.

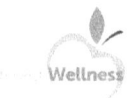

If you want to feel fabulous inside and out.

If you would like fabulous relationships.

If you would like to feel more connected, feel peace in your heart, and feel truly alive.

This program is different from any other weight loss and wellness program you have ever experienced in the past.

So how do we get started? First we have to ask, "Are you ready?" Well if you are reading this, you are at least considering some changes in your life. Awesome! This is the first step.

Our program starts with a 3-Phase approach, which is based on the paradigm of the stages of change.

**Stage 1 – Pre-contemplation**: you are unaware you have a problem or issues, in denial or just not in tune with your body or health.

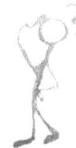

**Stage 2 – Contemplation**: you are aware of the problem and desire a behavior change. Maybe you don't feel well. Need to lose weight?

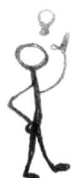

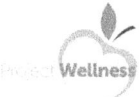

**Stage 3 – Preparation**: you intend to take action

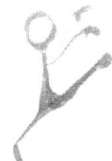

**Stage 4 – Action**: you begin "practicing" the desired behavior

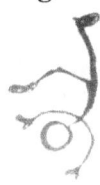

**Stage 5 – Maintenance**: you work to sustain the behavior change

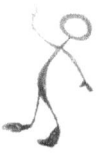

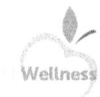

## Phase 1
### Pre-contemplation, Contemplation, and Preparation Phase

**Pre-contemplation** is the stage at which there is no intention to change behavior in the foreseeable future. Many individuals in this stage are unaware or under-aware of their problems. If you are reading this book, you want something different. You are AWARE! And this means you have taken the first step. If you have some vague intention to change, then you are moving into the next stage.

**Contemplation** is the stage in which people are aware that a problem exists and are seriously thinking about overcoming it, but have not yet made a commitment to take action. You may be here. You know that you are stressed out, overworked, burned out even, and are AWARE that a problem exists. We teach our patients that their health problems often have to get so great (this is often referred to as "rock-bottom") before they are ready to consider taking action. They stay in survival mode, not thriving mode, and keep doing the same thing expecting a different result.

**Preparation** is a stage that combines intention and behavioral criteria. Individuals in this stage are intending to take action in the next month and have unsuccessfully taken action in the past year. Maybe you have been looking at different options. Maybe even tried a few things that didn't work. They get scared. They go back to what they know. And this keeps you stuck. It always keeps you stuck. You have to release the fear and move into the action phase. Action phase is very important, and it is more important to have a game plan and a proven system to place your confidence in. If what you have done in the past doesn't work, don't keep doing it. If parts of it worked, learn from that experience, take those parts, and do the work to find the path that works. Find a mentor and ask the right questions. If you have done weight loss systems or joined gyms,

18

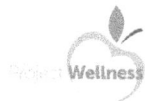 

they have probably been frustrating without a proven protocol or system that gives proven results. But you may have succeeded in some areas that may not have recognized. This is important. I tell my patients, "It was not one thing that caused you to be overweight, it was lots of things, so you can't just do one thing and expect sustainable results. You must have a systematic approach that addresses all the underlying issues".

That is what our system provides. It provides a system that when utilized and implemented addresses all the shortcomings and frustrations that you have met and brings you full circle so that you can maximize the best of everything that you have learned so far.

During this phase, we ask that you start changing your thoughts and your behaviors. We are working toward sustainable results, and the preparation stage is very important. Assessing your life, your behaviors, what is in your food pantry, and what your barriers may be are very important.

Remember this is a "marathon" for life and NOT a "sprint." If you take these changes slowly, they will be more sustainable. During this phase we ask that you start weaning off sodas, coffee, and sugary foods. We want you to start reading labels and become aware of what you are eating everyday. Gluten (protein in wheat) and dairy are major inflammatory food triggers, and we ask that you begin cutting them out. These are the only dietary restrictions that we ask you to start with.

If you have had food sensitivities done by blood work, these take about four weeks to get back, and then you will start on the 21-day detox (Phase 2). If you don't have a source for getting this done, we ask you to cut out the eight most common trigger foods for your detox.

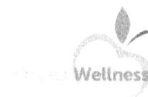
8 Food Sensitivities
These are the most common food sensitivities that we recommend you avoid during the detox.

**Corn**
**Eggs**
**Shellfish**
**Soy**
**Tomatoes**
**Cow's Milk/Dairy**
**Wheat/Gluten**
**Refined Sugar and artificial sweeteners**

## Phase 2
### 21-Day Detox
Specific eating plan (Project Nutrition Section) with substitutions for your food sensitivities. Begin exercise routine.

**Action** is the stage in which individuals modify their behavior, experiences, or environment in order to overcome their problems. Action involves the most overt behavioral changes and requires considerable commitment of time and energy. Embarking on this stage of the journey is the most overwhelming. It is when you are most likely to fall back into old patterns. You must have a system that is reproducible but INDIVIDUALIZED, because we are all different and have different engrained old un-healthy patterns and levels of "disease" in our psyche and physical bodies. We must first address where we fall short, what has worked in the past, and grow

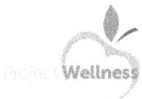

from all our experiences. We are all different with different needs, but the same basic principles apply.

---

**Phase 3**
**After The Detox**
Now starts the 3-Month rotation schedule according to your food sensitivities. This is considered your Maintenance phase. This time reinforces behaviors. We encourage education and empowerment through homework assignments and curriculum.

---

**Maintenance** is the stage in which people work to prevent relapse and consolidate the gains attained during action. For addictive behaviors, this stage extends from six months to an indeterminate period past the initial action. This is the phase that once you start to build confidence is vital to the long-term sustainable success that you seek. Working with a mentor or coach is so valuable during this phase because it allows you to make some mistakes while not sabotaging the long-term results by having someone that has been on that journey. They can reinforce that it is okay to make mistakes, and you just keep going. There will be mistakes. You will mess up. What you do with that decides your fate. You can fall into the "why me?" or victimized role or you can decide to make a different choice and move forward. Patients struggle the most in this phase. It is also during this phase when you may plateau with weight loss goals and start to feel frustrated. You may blame others and start to look for fault with the program you are on. You may start to look for something outside yourself that is keeping you from your goals. You may want to stop your forward progress. You may just give up hope like you have done in the past. Although you may see some results, you may really struggle when the "stress" sets in and relapses often occur. Having a coach or mentor can really solidify your resolve. Whatever choices you make find a coach to keep you on track.

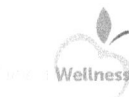

It is so hard for high-functioning people to ASK FOR HELP. I struggled with this for years. I thought I had to do it all by myself. It seemed like a sign of weakness to ask for help. I even found myself doing other's work, because it just seemed easier to do it than to ask them. Training is very important as well. Training is not the same as asking. Training requires work and it requires most importantly reinforcement. You must follow up and make sure that the program is first and foremost understood, but then implemented and sustained.

TRAIN-IMPLEMENT-TRAIN-IMPLEMENT-TRAIN-FOLLOW UP-TRAIN-IMPLEMENT-FOLLOW UP…. Until you are in maintenance phase, and then follow up some more!

As you make the decision to change your life, you will meet frustration and self-sabotaging behavior. Expect this! And ask for help!

Every day I get to do this and I feel so blessed and finally at peace that I am changing lives and doing the good that I always felt divinely compelled to do.

Are you ready to change your life? Change can be scary, but the results can be so rewarding. Keep your eye on the goal.

Know your goals!

Goal Setting

> **5 effective ways to achieve your goals**
> -Have a plan, and map out smaller sub-goals.
> -Tell your friends.
> -Remind yourself of the benefits of the reward. Focus on what you want, not what you don't want.
> -Reward yourself at sub-goals.
> -Write them down.

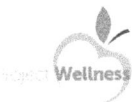

We like to refer to the "S.M.A.R.T." model of goal setting.

Create S.M.A.R.T. Goals

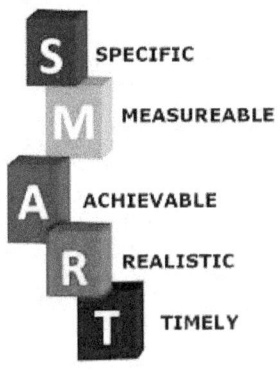

1. Specific goals for weight loss and wellness examples would be how much weight you want to lose. Don't just say, "I want to lose weight." Define how much you want to lose. "I want to be a size 8" would be a great example.
2. Measurable goals for weight loss would be, "I want to lose 50 pounds and I will lose 5 pounds per week."
3. Achievable goals are established based on where you are in your life. Have you lost 5 pounds per week in the past when all other variables were even? Can other people lose 5 pounds per week?
4. Realistic goals are within reason. It is not really reasonable to lose 50 pounds in 1 week.
5. Timely goals have a specific time frame in which to reach them. You may need to reevaluate at certain times to readjust the reality of the situation. Working with a coach or health care provider that can identify issues like inflammation, etc., can really help you reset your metabolism and get on track. One pitfall is to use time to frustrate you. If goals are not going according to the time frame, it's time to ask for help!

Objectives that probably don't work when goal-setting:

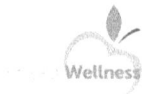
- Focusing only on someone successful.  There is only one "you," and your issues may be different than someone else's.

- Thinking about bad things that will happen if you don't reach your goal.  Focusing on the negative will only bring more of that into your life.

- Trying to suppress unhelpful thoughts (avoid thinking about unhealthy food or smoking).

- Relying on willpower.

Objectives that do work when goal-setting:

- Focusing on what you want to achieve.

- Thinking about the benefits of reaching your goal.  Ex.: I will feel better.  Enjoy shopping for new clothes, etc.  Visualize what it will feel like to feel good and be active.

- Embracing your deterring thoughts.  Understand that they have had their own benefits and have been protective on some level in the past. (i.e. comfort foods made you feel better…).  See section on stress.

- Relying on a specific plan of action.

4. Planning – moving forward.  What to expect next week.

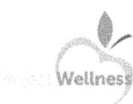

Who are the members of your support group (obtain names and emails)?

_____

_____

_____

What are my specific goals?

_____

_____

_____

What are the benefits of my goals?

_____

_____

_____

Who will I tell (pick a coach or supportive individual)?

_____

What am I committed to this week?

_____

All the while we are teaching healthy choices and tools for choosing behaviors that work with your individual lifestyle for sustainable results. Our team has years of experience in the area of how hormones influence weight loss and why most diets fail. We say, "We have cracked the weight loss code!"

When most people embark on wellness programs, diets, or losing weight, they often battle with feeling tired and hungry. The biggest benefit to Project Wellness followers is that they simply feel better, never feel hungry, and experience increased energy and vitality within the first 45 days of their program and working toward a balanced body. Close communication with a coach or mentor is vital to meeting the challenges that you may experience. These challenges are often the very obstacles that have kept you from your goals in the past. It is your responsibility to ask for help if you are not feeling well, meeting your goals, or experiencing self-sabotaging behaviors or setbacks. Patients in our program understand that we are responsible *to* you not *for* you. You must empower yourself and take action to identify your challenges so that you can get the help you need.

We encourage you to make the commitment to yourself to change your life forever by following all of the Project Wellness recommendations.

Our goal is that you make this investment for your health empowerment and embark on a journey of freedom from medications, illness, chronic disease, and dependence on the health care/medical system. Traditional medicine in our country is wonderful for acute illness, trauma, etc., but is just not positioned to promote your wellness and health goals. We congratulate you that you find the value in wellness and taking charge of your health. Insurance companies and pharmaceutical companies are just not conducive to your goals in this area. Your traditional doctors as well-meaning and well-trained as they are may not understand how we do what we do. You can share with them and others and in this process help educate everyone around you that there is a "different way"—a way of wellness and freedom from the traditional design of medicine in our country today. During the course of this book, we will take you on the journey to making changes in your life that are needed to "do something different." It has been said, "If you always do what you have always done, you will always get what you always got." We want to teach you to do something different to get a different result. The first four weeks we will explore who you are, what you want, and where you are going with your life and your goals. We will start you on your journey to eating "clean," making better decisions, introducing you to a discovery of motion of your body that will promote wellness (you may have labeled this as exercise in the past), and finding options that fit your individual lifestyle. The remainder of the weeks we will discuss how your

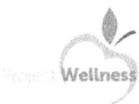
metabolism works, what your lab values mean, how to interpret them, and how we have a different approach that is very successful in balancing the system.

PHYSICAL INCLUDES THREE AREAS: MEDICAL, FITNESS, & NUTRITION

MEDICAL

**Why is lab screening & food allergies testing important to weight loss?**

To make an individualized program that will sustain you through the rest of your life, you need to understand how your body works and what metabolic imbalances look and feel like in correlation with your lab values and symptoms. It is essential to understanding what is going on in your body so that you can make the appropriate choices and changes.

Hormones

**What do hormones have to do with weight loss?**

Hormones have everything to do with every process in our bodies. Hormones go into the cell, insert themselves into your very DNA, and make proteins that tell the body what to do… this can be lose weight, gain weight, raise your metabolism, lower it, etc.

**What is included in most crucial lab screenings?**

We recommend a comprehensive weight loss hormone panel (including insulin, complete thyroid panel, and sex steroids: estrogen, testosterone, progesterone), nutritional test of B12, iron, vitamin D, cholesterol, complete blood count, and food sensitivities.

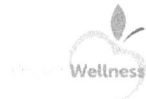

**What is included in the Food Allergy, sensitivity Testing and what do you test?**

This is a blood test of over 100 foods that trigger an immune response in your system. It is a delayed response by up to 3 days, so you may not even know that this food has triggered your immune system. Some people may feel fatigue, joint aches, or stomach upset. Some feel nothing but a general sense of inflammation often experienced as "bloating," and this may be in more than just the gastrointestinal tract.

**Why do you recommend a detox/cleanse?**

The detox has many aspects that prepare the gastrointestinal system for absorbing nutrients and restoring health in the body.

FITNESS

Why is fitness important to weight loss?

Our bodies were meant to be in motion. There is no substitute for dedicated movement. If you want to lose weight, you must burn fat. This can be done aerobically if the heart rate is up to target for a set amount of time or anaerobically by building muscle. Again, this is not a quick fix or magic pill, it is real physiological change with real psychological and emotional commitment.

Why is fitness an important part of the program?

Weight loss is a side effect of a balanced system. Our goal is complete balance. Fitness is a reflection of health, wellness, and balance.

Why is nutrition/food an important part of a health challenge?

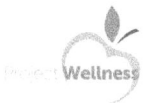

Learning to make healthy choices is our primary goal. Helping you understand not only the nutritional value of what you eat but also when and how you eat is very important as well. Without good nutrition, your body does not have the fuel it needs to optimize the processes that require balance.

MENTAL/EMOTIONAL

Why is mental/emotional a part of Project Wellness? Understanding "why we eat" is as important as "what we eat." Understanding stress as it relates to chronic disease and obesity is key to success. We teach understanding of stress in our behaviors and patterns by teaching the "Stress Model" and sharing the tools to overcome challenges day to day in weight loss and wellness, we bring the "why" out of you. Hold on to your seat as we break open the personal emotional blocks that have been standing in the way of you and success in life in all areas including your health. The first four weeks of the program are intense and life-changing.

Wellness

# Project Nutrition

### What to eat...

Why understand this?
How do you know you have food sensitivities?
What is leaky gut?
How to get started even before you have a blood test...8 trigger foods
Food allergy testing
Detox

Why understand nutrition?  Nutrition is just one pillar of a full comprehensive design for overall health and metabolic well-being, but it is an essential pillar.  Without any one pillar, the roof will fall, right?  We must begin to think in terms of food not as a social engagement but something that sustains life.  EAT TO LIVE!  Food is eaten to sustain life, provide energy, and promote growth and repair of tissues.

We must ask ourselves...do these do any of that?

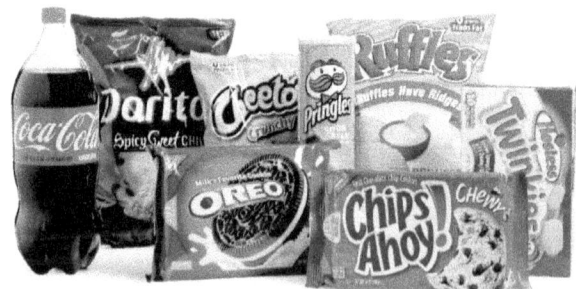

We all know the answer is no.  In fact, these are laden with chemicals that will deter growth, will drain our energy, and will deteriorate our tissues.

So, what if you are eating "HEALTHY?"

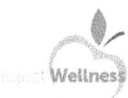

Well most people are eating "healthy" things they don't even know are literally making them fat. We had a movement in our country a few years ago to go "FAT FREE." We thought simply that "FAT" in foods must make us "FAT." Worse yet we thought that the fat in foods was causing cholesterol or fat in the blood and therefore heart and blood vessel issues leading to stroke and cardiovascular disease. We found that this wasn't true at all.

When people stopped eating a lot of fat, do you know what they ate more of? SUGAR!

We found that there was more obesity and more heart disease than ever. The sugar caused inflammation through insulin resistance and cortisol increases and adrenal exhaustion. We saw an increase in belly fat and diabetes. We were clearly very wrong.

So if that wasn't the answer, then what is? I have patients who try to decrease sugar or carbs and still gain weight or can't lose weight. Well I stumbled on to a very straightforward and interesting way to eat which is the basis for sustainable weight loss and wellness forever. Want to hear about it? Of course you do or you wouldn't be reading this.

Well there are foods that you may consider healthy but may not be right for you.

"But how do I know?" you might ask.

You probably don't know. But I will tell you not knowing is hurting you. Let me go into an analogy that one of our coaches shared with me.

Imagine you have a car and you have no idea what kind of gas it takes. You go to the pump and you look at the unleaded pump and the diesel fuel pump. Which one do you use? What if you guess and

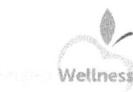

you are wrong? How far will your car go? If you put the wrong fuel in, what will be the fix? You have to have the pipes drained, right? Well, your body is no different. You might think certain foods are healthy, but they might not be the right fuel for you. And what do you do if you have the wrong fuel in your tank? This is the basis for understanding food sensitivities and detox.

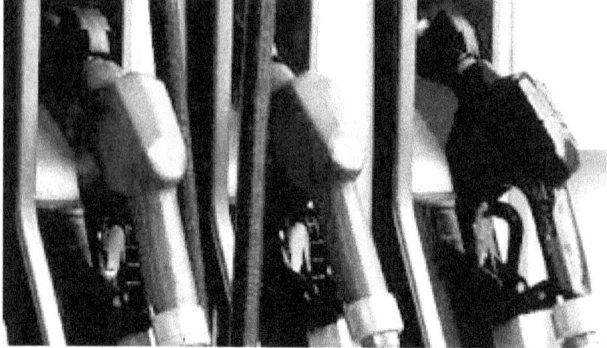

But first, let me ask you,

**Are you experiencing...**

1. Digestive issues such as gas, bloating, diarrhea or irritable bowel syndrome (IBS)?
2. Seasonal allergies or asthma?
3. Hormonal imbalances such as menopause symptoms, heavy periods, endometriosis, PMS, or PCOS? Low libido? Hot flashes?
4. Diagnosis of an autoimmune disease such as rheumatoid arthritis, Hashimoto's thyroiditis, lupus, psoriasis, or celiac disease?
5. Fatigue?
6. Chronic fatigue?
7. Fibromyalgia? Hurt all the time for no apparent reason?
8. Mood and mind issues such as depression, anxiety, attention deficit issues?
9. Skin issues such as acne, rosacea, or eczema? Itching
10. Diagnosis of yeast infections, or food allergies or intolerances?
11. Memory loss?
12. Cancer, aging, or heart disease?

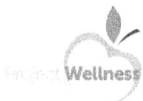
If you said yes to any of these, you probably have food sensitivities.

Before we talk about food sensitivities, we need to discuss a controversial topic that is very pertinent to our discussion called "Leaky Gut"!

## What is… LEAKY GUT

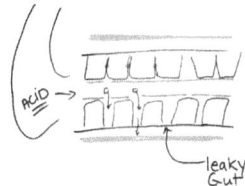

**Normal Intestines**          **Leaky Intestines**

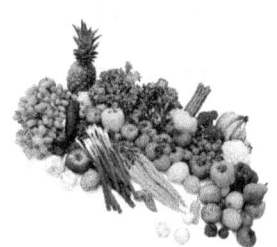

Even if you ate veggies from the Garden of Eden, organic and rich with nutrients, you would still have to have a perfectly healthy digestive tract, stomach, and intestine, to absorb the nutrients from it that you need. The intestine or gut is naturally permeable to very small molecules in order to absorb these vital nutrients. In fact, regulating intestinal permeability is one of the basic functions of the cells that line the intestinal wall. In sensitive people, gluten can cause the gut cells to release "Zonulin," a protein that can break apart tight junctions in the intestinal lining. Other factors—such as infections, toxins, stress, and age—can also cause these tight junctions to break apart.

Once these tight junctions get broken apart, you have a leaky gut. When your gut is leaky, things like toxins, microbes, undigested food particles, and more can escape from your intestines and travel throughout your body via your bloodstream. Your immune system marks these "foreign invaders" as pathogens and attacks them.

So, **what causes leaky gut?**

The main culprits are foods, infections, toxins, and gluten, a protein found in wheat, inflammatory foods like dairy, or toxic foods, such as sugar and excessive alcohol. The most common infectious causes are yeast, intestinal parasites, and small intestine bacterial overgrowth. Toxins come in the form of medications, like Motrin, Advil, steroids, antibiotics, and acid-reducing drugs, and environmental toxins like mercury, pesticides, and BPA from plastics. Stress, leaking stomach acid into the intestines, hormone changes and age also contribute to a leaky gut.

The good news is there's a solution to healing leaky gut. To keep it simple, here are some basics to start with…

1. Remove foods and factors that damage the gut such as sugar, grains, dairy, GMO foods, non-organic foods, acidic substances like coffee, drugs like ibuprofen, acid reducers, and non-essential antibiotics. Ask your doctor about medications that you may not need. **Get food allergy testing!** Identify your specific food sensitivities and remove them from your diet. A 21-day detox protocol of eliminating the foods you are sensitive to is

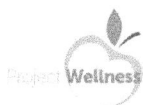

essential to healing the gut. If your car had diesel fuel in it and it was an unleaded gas engine, you would need to remove the wrong fuel from the line.

2. Replace with healing foods like Bone Broth, Fermented Vegetables, Coconut, and Super seeds like chia seeds, flaxseeds, and hemp seeds (as long as they are not on your food sensitivity/allergy list). Also, consuming foods that have anti-inflammatory Omega-3 fats are beneficial such as grass-fed beef, lamb, and wild caught fish like salmon.

3. Repair with specific supplements, these include specific amino acids, magnesium, digestive enzymes, pro-biotics and anti-inflammatories. Certain amino acids act like "gut spackling" and protects and coats the intestinal wall, and acts as an anti-inflammatory as well as does Aloe Vera licorice, Reservatrol, and Turmeric among many others we recommend. Digestive enzymes ensure that food is fully digested, decreasing the chance of undigested foods traversing the leaky gut and causing immune response. Magnesium relaxes smooth muscle in the gut, keeping things moving.

4. Rebalance with probiotics. Last but most important, this is THE Vital Part to Healing Your Gut. You must rebalance with the right probiotics. Many on the market have the wrong ratio or have ingredients that may make your issues worse. It is essential to get at least 100 billion units the right ratio of bacteria.

If you can follow the above protocol, you are well on your way to healing your gut for good!

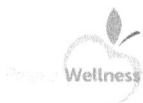
Leaky Gut:

The inability to absorb vital nutrients can cause imbalances in the system.

Food allergy/sensitivity testing is a vital piece to the balance that the system is seeking as well as supplements that heal the digestive process.

### Food Allergy/Sensitivity
### A powerful tool for your weight loss and wellness program

**What is food sensitivity?**

When I first learned about food sensitivities, I was working with a chiropractor. He was using food sensitivities for joint pain, chronic pain, fibromyalgia, and all the maladies that most patients seek out a chiropractor for. I have always been amazed at how chiropractors know things that traditional doctors don't. They don't have a prescription pad at their fingertips, so they have to learn what "works" if they really want to get results. He taught me the basics of how certain foods trigger inflammation in the body and how this inflammation spreads to joints, muscles, and tendons causing pain. But more than that, this inflammation is in the blood vessels and causing more insidious disease that may end in heart disease, strokes, cancer, autoimmune disease, and possible cancer. These end points resulting in possible death. I watched as he ordered test after test and got amazing results.

I had a patient who came in one day with obvious hormone imbalance and terrible fibromyalgia. I was thinking it was the hormone imbalance but after I clearly corrected that, she still continued to have pain. So I did what my chiropractor friend recommended and ordered the food sensitivity test.

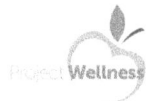

She returned for the results, and I explained how it worked. She seemed skeptical, and we scheduled her a three-month follow up appointment.

I watched her walk into the room without limping, without her cane, and without obvious distress. She had a glow about her that I could not explain. Her skin was brighter and her mood lighter. She took a seat, and although her physical state was remarkably improved, she had an energy about her that was confusing. She smiled softly. I noticed that she appeared about twenty pounds lighter than I had seen her last.

"Looks like you are doing much better!" I exclaimed.

"Oh, I am… but…"

"But what?!?" I looked puzzled.

"I am doing amazing. I have lost twenty pounds. My joints do not hurt and the muscle pain is ninety percent improved. I have followed the food sensitivity test and had remarkable results. I am quite upset, however."

"Go on," I encouraged her.

"I am very frustrated because over six years ago, a doctor did the food sensitivity test on me and recommended that I make dietary changes. I thought he was crazy. I'm upset because I have suffered for over six years with these symptoms and the answer was so simple. Right in front of me! It took you with your confidence to convince me, or maybe just the tremendous suffering to finally take the leap and make some changes. I am so grateful for the change in my life but frustrated that I didn't listen sooner and I have suffered so much all these years."

I was amazed as she told me this and I took this to heart. I started using the test on everyone that I could think of with chronic pain. I never really thought about the weight loss as I thought that was just an effect of her eating less.

A few years and many patient success stories later, all the while not acknowledging the effects of the weight loss, I had a husband and wife come in the office one day. He was having terrible gastrointestinal symptoms. His wife was very frustrated and felt that it was affecting his health. He had terrible gas, bloating, and constipation alternating with diarrhea every time he ate. He had been diagnosed with "IBS" or irritable bowel syndrome and put on many prescription medications that simply did not help. It was affecting his work, his home life, and his sleep. He was in terrible pain all over and his hormones were all out of balance by blood test. I recommended the food sensitivity test.

He was more than willing to comply as no one had helped him thus far. We discussed dietary substitutions and he returned for his follow up three months later. He was thrilled. He had lost thirty pounds and he was so happy to be empowered to know what foods caused his pain and distress. He had avoided them strictly and adhered to the recommendations. All was well… Or so I thought. His wife was quite upset. She sat in the opposite chair with a very closed off energy, her arms crossed about her chest, and a stern look on her face. I turned to her and said, "Aren't you happy that he is doing so well?"

"Oh, yes!" She replied. "He is doing great, but since I have been cooking for him, I have gained twenty pounds!"

I was confused. "How could cooking for him, the clean and healthy foods that I recommended while avoiding his trigger foods have caused her to gain weight? Was something else going on?" And

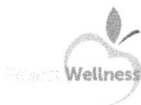 

then I realized that maybe there was a recurring theme to this weight loss I had witnessed in patients who had complied with the dietary recommendations. Maybe hers were different? And so I recommended that we test her, to which she was reluctant but agreed.

To my amazement, her list of foods that she was sensitive too was almost completely opposite of his. I realized in that moment the power of this food sensitivity program. She was willing to try to make meals separately for each of them, and at her three month follow-up, she had lost the extra twenty she had gained plus ten more pounds. "Holy crap!" I thought. "This is huge!"

I had personally gained almost eighty pounds on synthetic hormones after my hysterectomy, and when I went on bio-identical hormones and started exercising, I had lost all but the last fifteen or twenty pounds. I thought to myself that I would do the test and see if this really worked. So I did… *and it did!* I am down to 130 pounds and follow my list very closely and feel wonderful. Years of stomach pain and IBS and struggling with my weight were gone. I have since used this strategy on thousands of patients and get consistent results as long as the patient understands, believes, and adheres to the test and follows it. I had been giddy with the discovery until I went to my annual continuing education courses at the anti-aging conference and learned that many doctors all over the world are using the food sensitivity results for weight loss. I had patted myself on the back for discovering this and felt quite deflated in that I did not really discover anything at all.

We have created a whole program around food sensitivities and continue to get incredible results.

"So how does this work?" you may ask.

The inability to tolerate certain foods, also known as insensitivity or intolerance, induces chronic activation of the immune system. Free

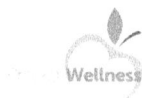

radicals and mediators of inflammation are produced. This inflammation has been linked to countless chronic conditions including: digestive disorders, migraines, obesity, chronic fatigue, attention deficit issues, aching joints, skin disorders, arthritis, and many more.

This inflammation induces a cortisol response from the adrenal glands, which ultimately leads to unwanted belly fat. See section on hormones.

**How does food sensitivity differ from classic food allergies?**

True or immediate food allergies refer to foods that trigger the immune system to acutely produce massive amounts of the chemical histamine that leads to anaphylaxis or a potentially fatal condition that may cause the throat and esophagus (swallowing tube) to swell, cutting off air from the lungs, or may simply cause hives, skin rashes, and other non-life-threatening reactions.

This type of reaction is called a hypersensitivity reaction, caused by the degranulation of mast cells or basophils that is mediated by Immunoglobulin E (IgE). This happens within minutes.

Then there is a delayed reaction that can take up to 3 days to appear. This is mediated by the part of the immune system called IgG.

Food allergies are divided into two major categories: immediate and delayed. Delayed can take up to 72 hours to appear.

Some people get confused about food allergies versus sensitivities. When we talk of the delayed response, we often refer to this as a "sensitivity" or "food intolerance."

Non-IgE-mediated food hypersensitivity (food intolerance) is more chronic, less acute, less obvious in its presentation, and often more difficult to diagnose than a food allergy. Symptoms of food

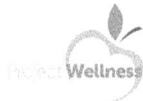
intolerance vary greatly, and can be mistaken for the symptoms of a food allergy.

While true allergies are associated with fast-acting immunoglobulin IgE responses, it can be difficult to determine the offending food, causing a food intolerance because the response generally takes place over a prolonged period of time. Thus, the causative agent and the response are separated in time and may not be obviously related. Food intolerance symptoms usually begin about half an hour after eating or drinking the food in question, but sometimes symptoms may be delayed up to 48 hours.

Food intolerance can present with symptoms affecting the skin, respiratory tract, or gastrointestinal tract, either individually or in combination. On the skin, it may include skin rashes, itching, hives, swelling, and chronic eczema. Respiratory tract symptoms can include a stuffy nose, sinus infections, asthma, and cough among many. Gastrointestinal symptoms may include ulcers in the mouth, reflux, or chest pain (heart burn), abdominal cramps, nausea, gas, bloating, intermittent diarrhea or constipation (irritable bowel symptoms-IBS), and vomiting or even prolonged gastritis, bleeding, hemorrhoids, ulcers, and chronic gastrointestinal pain.

Other symptoms include headaches and joint and muscle pains and lead to more insidious disease from the inflammation like cancer, aging, and cardiovascular disease (heart attacks and strokes).

So if you have any symptoms, there are a couple things you can do to test to see if you have food sensitivities.

FIFTEEN/FIFTEEN Rule: One quick and dirty test you can do is to get a stop-watch and monitor your pulse for one minute. If you eat something you are sensitive to, your pulse will go up fifteen or more beats within fifteen minutes. The problem with this is that it is sensitive but not specific. You won't know what food triggered you. If you eat multiple foods, it could be any one of them. You can

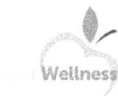

experiment with different isolated foods to do this test. The problem is that it has to be a pretty severe sensitivity to trigger a response this quickly. Some of the milder triggers may take up to three days to trigger this response.

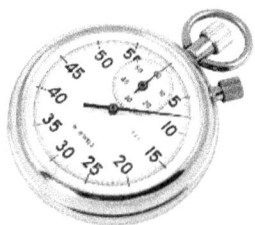

One other way you can try is the elimination diet, but this can be tricky because often when someone gives up one food, they eat more of something else they could be triggered by.

The other much more reasonable option is just to have your blood tested. This is sensitive and specific and spot-on every time.

How do you test for them?

This is measured as IgG, unlike IgE (immediate response/allergy). This is a delayed response by the immune system. To verify if you have an IgG food intolerance, a simple blood test can be done to identify 100 to 200 foods. The test examines the blood directly. A blood sample is taken, the lab technician identifies delayed onset allergies by observing how white blood cells and red blood cells react if they are exposed to selected foods. Red and white blood cell samples literally explode when allergens are introduced. What is also excellent about the allergy test is that the test will not be tied to detecting food intolerances; it may also identify reactions to artificial additives, antibiotics, environmental chemicals, and pharmacological ingredients.

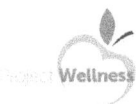

The process measures the amount of response as well as if there is a response of your white blood cell antibodies (IgG) to protein substance (antigens) in the specific foods tested.

| IgE | IgA and IgG |
|---|---|
| Fast response (few minutes) | Slower response (2 hours-72 hours), sometimes take years for symptoms to manifest |
| Strong response | Weaker response |
| Similar physiological response in most people | Varied physiological response in most people |
| "fixed"- do not change during our lifetime | Can evolve at any age |
| Analogous to immune system "blow-torch": instant, acute, powerful | Analogous to immune system "sand paper": delayed, slowly damaging |
| Immune system response to a protein found in digestive system that is perceived as foreign object | Immune system response to a protein found in digestive system that is perceived as foreign object |

This is a sample food allergy test panel from Alletess, the company we use most often.

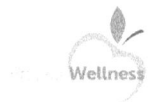

| TEST | SCORE | CLASS | | TEST | SCORE | CLASS | |
|---|---|---|---|---|---|---|---|
| ALMOND | 0.179 | 0 | | LETTUCE | 0.158 | 0 | |
| APPLE | 0.159 | 0 | | LOBSTER | 0.170 | 0 | |
| ASPARAGUS | 0.175 | 0 | | MALT | 0.157 | 0 | |
| AVOCADO | 0.157 | 0 | | MILK (COW'S) | 0.310 | 2 | ** |
| BANANA | 0.161 | 0 | | MUSHROOM | 0.211 | 1 | * |
| BARLEY | 0.263 | 1 | * | MUSTARD | 0.168 | 0 | |
| BASIL | 0.170 | 0 | | NUTRA SWEET | 0.157 | 0 | |
| BAY LEAF | 0.160 | 0 | | OAT | 0.166 | 0 | |
| BEAN (GREEN) | 0.172 | 0 | | OLIVE (GREEN) | 0.155 | 0 | |
| BEAN (LIMA) | 0.176 | 0 | | ONION | 0.161 | 0 | |
| BEAN (PINTO) | 0.289 | 1 | * | ORANGE | 0.172 | 0 | |
| BEEF | 0.168 | 0 | | OREGANO | 0.155 | 0 | |
| BLUEBERRY | 0.150 | 0 | | PEA | 0.182 | 0 | |
| BRAN | 0.155 | 0 | | PEACH | 0.148 | 0 | |
| BROCCOLI | 0.222 | 1 | * | PEANUT | 0.151 | 0 | |
| CABBAGE | 0.163 | 0 | | PEAR | 0.139 | 0 | |
| CANTALOUPE | 0.190 | 0 | | PEPPER (BLACK) | 0.151 | 0 | |
| CARROT | 0.172 | 0 | | PEPPER (CHILI) | 0.153 | 0 | |
| CASHEW | 0.213 | 1 | * | PEPPER (GREEN) | 0.151 | 0 | |
| CAULIFLOWER | 0.206 | 1 | * | PINEAPPLE | 0.266 | 1 | * |
| CELERY | 0.149 | 0 | | PORK | 0.127 | 0 | |
| CHEESE (CHEDDAR) | 0.144 | 0 | | POTATO (SWEET) | 0.145 | 0 | |
| CHEESE (COTTAGE) | 0.141 | 0 | | POTATO (WHITE) | 0.147 | 0 | |
| CHEESE (SWISS) | 0.146 | 0 | | RICE | 0.137 | 0 | |
| CHICKEN | 0.155 | 0 | | RYE | 0.206 | 1 | * |
| CINNAMON | 0.122 | 0 | | SAFFLOWER | 0.149 | 0 | |
| CLAM | 0.139 | 0 | | SALMON | 0.184 | 0 | |
| COCOA | 0.209 | 1 | * | SCALLOP | 0.146 | 0 | |
| COCONUT | 0.173 | 0 | | SESAME | 0.139 | 0 | |
| CODFISH | 0.151 | 0 | | SHRIMP | 0.159 | 0 | |
| COFFEE | 0.266 | 1 | * | SOLE | 0.190 | 0 | |
| COLA | 0.144 | 0 | | SOYBEAN | 0.144 | 0 | |
| CORN | 0.141 | 0 | | SPINACH | 0.143 | 0 | |
| CRAB | 0.231 | 1 | * | SQUASH | 0.145 | 0 | |
| CUCUMBER | 0.159 | 0 | | STRAWBERRY | 0.142 | 0 | |
| DILL | 0.151 | 0 | | SUGAR (CANE) | 0.134 | 0 | |
| EGG WHITE | 0.290 | 1 | * | SUNFLOWER (SEED) | 0.136 | 0 | |
| EGG YOLK | 0.193 | 0 | | SWORDFISH | 0.147 | 0 | |
| EGGPLANT | 0.161 | 0 | | TEA (BLACK) | 0.163 | 0 | |
| GARLIC | 0.141 | 0 | | TOMATO | 0.156 | 0 | |
| GINGER | 0.256 | 1 | * | TUNA | 0.200 | 1 | * |
| GLUTEN | 0.319 | 2 | ** | TURKEY | 0.151 | 0 | |
| GRAPE | 0.150 | 0 | | WALNUT (BLACK) | 0.166 | 0 | |
| GRAPEFRUIT | 0.161 | 0 | | WATERMELON | 0.162 | 0 | |
| HADDOCK | 0.147 | 0 | | WHEAT | 0.310 | 2 | ** |

You can see on this test that the foods in red have triggered an IgG reaction in this patient and it is rated 1, 2, or 3. The higher the number the more reactive the patient is to that food. 3 is the worst— the higher the number, the worse the reaction.

During your detox, you avoid all foods in red, and afterward, in the rotation schedule, you rotate foods with a 1 or 2 every 3-5 days and avoid 3's. The rationale for this is that it takes approximately 3 days to develop a new IgG antibody/antigen protein reaction, giving your body time to reset the inflammatory response.

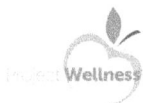

How do I proceed with my new diet? How do I know if ingredients are present in prepackaged foods that I eat? This is a sample of an ingredient label. You must read all labels very carefully. Even things that you would not suspect like vitamins and supplements may contain foods that you may be sensitive to. You have to read all labels. I was watching a show on the Discovery Channel where they were making sausage and they were putting gluten in it to make it look like more food. They call these fillers or thickeners. Even cosmetics may have foods that you are sensitive to. The ingredient list on a food label is the listing of each ingredient in descending order of predominance.

## Healing the Intestinal Tract

This is one of the most important aspects of true sustainable health. It's not what most people think and in the line of thinking to "do something different" this is one of the most critical steps.

The goal is to heal the intestinal tract aka "the gut" and once the gut is healed you are on your wait to sustainable weight loss, improved health, eliminating autoimmune disorders and regaining balance of your hormones.

EEK! Do you feel your best???? If not read on....

Considering that chronic diseases such as diabetes, autoimmunity, and liver failure, as well as common symptoms, like eczema, anxiety, fatigue, weight gain, bloating, and muscle/joint pain, can all be caused by leaky gut syndrome (otherwise known as LGS or intestinal permeability), it is imperative that you determine whether it may be occurring in your body.

Leaky gut is not well recognized by most practitioners, and is not found with the usual tests, not even with an endoscopy or colonoscopy. Still, there are close to 11,000 research studies about intestinal permeability from the past sixty years that clearly indicate that this is real health issue, including 35 studies released in just the past month.

For many, identifying leaky gut can be life changing because it is a condition that can be addressed with diet changes, nutrients, herbs, enzymes, and probiotics that help the intestinal lining to heal. In a medical system where people often find themselves reliant on medications, it is empowering to discover that there are natural solutions to address not only leaky gut, but challenging health concerns throughout their body.

I want to help you to know whether leaky gut could be an issue for you, so I've sorted through the research and pulled out the top reasons to think that you might have leaky gut.

Tired, Achy, Bloated, and/or Anxious?

While leaky gut can cause digestive troubles such as IBS, diarrhea, bloating, heartburn and stomach pain, it is quite possible that you won't experience any digestive distress at all. Instead, it is more common to feel worn out, in pain (anywhere in your body), and/or experience anxiety, depression or feel full of worry. That's because when the gut is leaky, it is like having tiny holes in your intestinal lining. Undigested food travels through these holes and into the underlying space where it triggers the immune system to try and protect you by launching an attack on the pieces of food that shouldn't be there.

These are some of the primary issues that may show up to make you think you have leaky gut.

1. Seasonal allergies or asthma.

2. Hormonal imbalances such as PMS or PCOS.

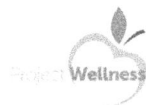

3. Diagnosis of an autoimmune disease such as rheumatoid arthritis, Hashimoto's thyroiditis, lupus, psoriasis, or celiac disease.

4. Diagnosis of chronic fatigue or fibromyalgia.

5. Mood and mind issues such as depression, anxiety, ADD or ADHD.

6. Skin issues such as acne, rosacea, or eczema.

7. Diagnosis of yeast or candida overgrowth.

8. Food allergies or food intolerances. Celiac or gluten intolerance.

This process results in the release of many inflammatory messengers (cytokines and antibodies) that lead to fatigue (even chronic fatigue syndrome), achiness (such as migraines, fibromyalgia and arthritis), allergies (on the skin like eczema, and in the sinuses and lungs, like asthma), and anxiety (which is known to be caused by inflammation in the nervous system), amongst other issues (see below).

Leaky gut also stresses the adrenal glands, making adrenal burnout more likely. It disrupts other hormones in the body as well, leading to PMS, menstrual irregularities, and breast and uterine issues. Over or under weight, as well as high or low cholesterol, and blood sugar issues

That's right, leaky gut can cause you to gain weight—for a few possible reasons. It is well cited in recent research that leaky gut increases the likelihood of insulin resistance (when insulin is not able to move sugar into your cells and leaves you with elevated blood sugar levels) and diabetes.
This occurs especially in combination with an imbalance in the healthy bacteria that should be living in our intestines. It appears that

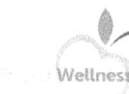
having too few healthy bacteria, along with permeability in the intestinal lining—and the inflammation that results—makes it more likely that your carbohydrate metabolism will be overwhelmed due to decreased insulin function, leading to weight gain. Any time carbohydrates are not able to make it into your cells (due to low insulin function), the body puts the excess carbs/sugar into storage as fat in your liver (which can lead to liver failure) or as cholesterol in your blood instead.

At the same time, an increasing number of fat cells release more of a hormone called leptin, which can lead to a disruption in the signals that you make you feel hungry and full. Before long, it can cause you to feel hungry even when you just ate, leading you to consume more calories than your body can possibly use.
For others, leaky gut results in difficulty gaining weight. That often occurs when there are digestive issues such as nausea, heartburn, and/or diarrhea that lead to a struggle to find foods you can consume without feeling worse. It also occurs because nutrients are not well absorbed when the gut is leaky. It is the job of the cells lining the intestine to digest and absorb nutrients. When these cells are damaged, they are not able to complete this function and nutrient depletion results.

Autoimmunity

If you have been diagnosed with any type of autoimmunity, that is a reason to think that you have may leaky gut. Research has confirmed that leaky gut is involved in the development of autoimmunity. The current theory is that when the spaces between the intestinal cells (called tight junctions) are open—which is the case with leaky gut— then the immune system begins to react to substances that it usually would not attack, including food and healthy cells.
In the case of celiac disease, the immune system begins attacking an enzyme that helps to repair the tight junctions. Other types of autoimmune conditions could result instead, such as Hashimoto's thyroiditis, lupus, MS, and/or rheumatoid arthritis. Genetic research

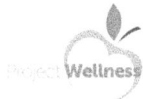

is helping us understand that, while the type of autoimmune condition that develops is genetically determined, it is leaky gut that gets the process started.

Use of antacids, anti-inflammatory drugs and/or antibiotics

Sometimes they are necessary, for a period of time, but overuse or extended use of antacids (for reflux or heartburn), anti-inflammatory drugs (for pain) and/or antibiotics (for infections) is known to cause leaky gut.
Antacids cause leaky gut by suppressing digestion of your food, making it more likely that your immune system will be triggered by the food you eat. Once the immune system starts to react, leaky gut is aggravated each time you eat, even if it is a food that you would think is good for you. The best way to get ahead is to figure out which foods are making things worse, so you can avoid them. How? Start by doing an IgG and IgA food sensitivity panel before you even begin treating the leaky gut itself. Gluten, found in bread, pasta, and pastries, is known to cause leaky gut, and so even if you don't yet have a food sensitivity panel, you can start by eliminating gluten from your diet.

Anti-inflammatory drugs (NSAIDS, Aleve, Advil, and Motrin) directly inflame the intestinal lining which also causes leaky gut. Antibiotics destroy the balance of healthy bacteria, which itself causes leaky gut, but also predispose you to the overgrowth of candida/yeast and unhealthy bacteria, that also lead to leaky gut. Healthy bacteria are important for making nutrients and processing toxins, but in their absence nutrient deficiency and toxicity results, making it more difficult for your colon and liver to stay healthy. Read more about the importance of healthy bacteria here.
All of this leads to a vicious cycle. The more you take these medications, the more leaky gut increases and the more pain, infections, and digestive upset you experience. It can seem like the only solution is to take medication. The real solution is to heal the leaky gut, decrease the pain and inflammation, and help your body

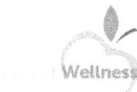
fight off infections naturally—preventing the need for the medications that create the vicious cycle.

Over-stressed?

Stress, in all its forms, has been shown to cause leaky gut. Stress also disrupts the balance of healthy bacteria in the gut, which further promotes leaky gut. Toxins in our food, water and environment (such as from pesticides in food, carpets in your home and exhaust fumes on the highway) also put stress on our systems that results in leaky gut. Gluten, as mentioned above, causes leaky gut by increasing levels of a protein called zonulin, which opens up the spaces between the intestinal cells, even if you don't have gluten sensitivity.

If you have been emotionally stressed on top of being exposed to gluten, pesticides, and/or heavy metals (in water and dental fillings), it is quite likely that you have at least some degree of leaky gut.

How to Find Out For Sure If You Have Leaky Gut
There are several tests that have been developed, and more on the way, that can tell you if you have some degree of leaky gut.

It is also possible to identify leaky gut by checking for IgG and IgA antibodies to food in a blood test – and this test is often preferable because it gives us two pieces of information:
Whether or not there is leaky gut; and
Which foods you can avoid to help heal the leaky gut (if it's there).

Note: Leaky gut cannot be found with an endoscopy or colonoscopy, and does not show on standard blood work, so it is missed by most practitioners.

The first step is to repair the gut and during this time, the first step is to avoid your food sensitivities.  If you have not had food sensitivities done then we recommend that you still do the

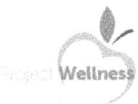

detoxification program as outlined below, avoiding the 8 most common food sensitivities.

During this time we recommend that you heal the gut with supplements that heal the intestinal tract. We have a few companies that we recommend.

# Project Detox

## Detoxification Protocol Program

Finding out your food sensitivities is a wonderful gift! You now know the right fuel to put in your tank! You will never be the same again. Though you may be shocked and scared when you first see the list (this is normal, everyone reacts with a little shock and fear), you will now know what you need to know to begin changing your life, reducing inflammation, and preventing disease due to inflammation. You are going to receive an abundance of wonderful and healthful benefits throughout the completion of your journey to wellness. A new YOU is waiting. We are going to reach your goals and meet that new YOU together!

The next step is the detoxification process and is outlined below. This is to cleanse the liver and digestive system, allowing your body to function at its fullest.

We hope you will find this protocol easy to understand and follow.

You are going to quickly realize that we do things differently at Project Wellness. Our goal is to be extraordinary! Prepare yourself for a wonderful journey to a lifetime of health, vitality, and wellness. Prepare to RECLAIM YOUR LIFE!

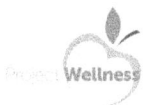

## **Detoxification**

The following diet plan is a sample plan. It is designed to avoid the BIG 8 food sensitivities. It should be followed as closely as possible. It is important that you avoid the foods that are on your food sensitivity list and take in the proteins, carbohydrates, and fats as suggested. However, it can be altered and "moved around" to fit your needs. Be diligent, take control of your health, and enjoy the benefits.

Once you have completed the detoxification program, you will be able to start adding the foods that are 1's and 2's back into your diet on a rotation schedule.

Protein supplementation is a vital part of your Project Wellness program. During the detoxification phase, we ask that you use a specific type of protein for your program and lifestyle. The type of protein we now recommend to all of our patients is a high quality Brown Rice protein powder supplement. We recommend brown rice protein as it is easily digested and utilized. Brown rice protein does not cause any digestive or side effect issues like we see with Whey or Casein type protein supplements.

Once you have completed your detoxification, you may switch to our high quality whey protein. If you begin to notice digestive side effects, you may want to consider returning to the rice protein.

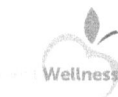

# Sample Grocery List

(Remember: shop according to your food sensitivity list if you tested)

Filtered Water 3-6 gallons (See desired amount to drink from chart above)
Fresh Limes and/or Lemons
Organic Maple Syrup-Grade B
Green Tea
Protein Drink (Vegetable: Pea or Rice)
Herbal Tea
Turkey Breast (Organic if possible)
Chicken Breast  (Organic if possible)
Fish-Tilapia, Salmon, Tuna, etc.
Fresh fruit: Apples, pears, melons, berries, peaches, nectarines, kiwi, citrus. No bananas or mango.
Almonds (Raw nuts and seeds are best)
Cashews
Sunflower seeds
Pumpkin seeds
Green vegetables
Salad Greens
Spinach
Broccoli
Cauliflower
Squash
Zucchini
Carrots
Onion
Garlic
Potato
Sweet Potato
Beans
Peas
French Vinaigrette Dressing or other suitable oil based dressing
Olive oil
Brown Rice
Rice Crackers
Organic Almond Butter or Cashew Butter
Spices of any kind are acceptable for cooking
Steel Cut Oats

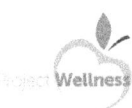

**21 DAY DETOXIFICATION PROTOCOL** – Remember if you have had food sensitivity testing to substitute any foods that you are sensitive to.

## PREPARATION PHASE 1 - SAMPLE MENU  - *DAYS 1 TO 8*

**Breakfast**
Protein Shake,　　 1 serving before breakfast
1 serving: Turkey or Chicken
OR 1 serving: Steel Cut Oatmeal or Gluten Free Rolled Oats (may use 1 packet of Stevia to sweeten) and 1 serving: Fresh Fruit (Stick with berries or pitted fruit)

**Morning Snack**
(Not mandatory) Nuts, animal protein and/or protein supplement shake

**Lunch**
Fresh green or spinach salad with olive oil dressing (You can use this throughout the program)
Fish – broiled or baked
Steamed/ raw/grilled/baked vegetables

**Afternoon Snack**
(Not mandatory) Nuts, animal protein and/or protein supplement shake

**Dinner**
1 serving: Turkey or Chicken Breast or Fish—broiled/steamed/raw/grilled/baked—vegetables, beans or peas, salad

**Nighttime Snack**
(Not mandatory) vegetable, almond butter, or small protein shake

## FOODS TO EAT DURING THIS PHASE
Drink plenty of fresh water (8-10 glasses), herbal teas, green tea
Eat as much fresh cruciferous vegetables as you want (again watching your food sensitivities)
Grain foods from rice, millet, quinoa, buckwheat, tapioca
Fresh fruits, vegetables, beans, peas

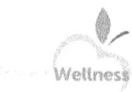
Fish, chicken, turkey *if* cold cuts-> (To truly detoxify Eat only organic: **no** additives/nitrates/nitrites/growth hormones/MSG/preservatives

Olive oil, flaxseed oil, coconut oil, all natural seasonings, sea salt

## FOODS TO AVOID DURING THIS PHASE

Any food that you know you are allergic/sensitive

Dairy (milk, cheeses, yogurt, butter), eggs, margarine, shortening

Foods prepared with Gluten-containing cereals like wheat, oats, rye, barley, those ingredients normally found in breads, pasta, etc.

Tomatoes and tomato sauces, corn (GMO), peanuts

Alcohol, caffeine (coffee, black tea, soda), sweeteners

Soy products, beef, pork, conventional cold cuts (Oscar Mayer), bacon, hotdogs, canned meat, sausage, shellfish, meat substitutes, shellfish

Fried food, dried fruit, or fruit juices

## DETOXIFICATION PHASE 2-SAMPLE MENU - *DAYS 8 TO 14* (No animal protein)

Note: This phase is important to remove animal protein from the diet for allowing the liver and system to reset. It can be a difficult time for fatigue and setbacks. But it is very important. We recommend that you do this every 3-6 months to detoxify the system.

**Breakfast**          Protein Shake 1 serving before breakfast
                       Steel Cut Oatmeal & Fruit or Gluten Free Rolled Oats

**Morning Snack**      Carrot sticks or celery & protein shake

Protein Shake,   1 serving before lunch

**Lunch**              Salad with nuts, seeds, avocado/Olive Oil Dressing

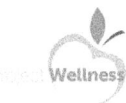

Steamed/raw/grilled/baked vegetables

**Afternoon Snack**     Fresh fruit or nuts & protein shake

**Dinner**     Protein Shake, 1 serving before dinner
Baked Potato or Baked Sweet Potato
Brown rice & Steamed/raw/grilled/baked
vegetables, beans, peas
Salad

**Nighttime Snack**     (Not mandatory) vegetable, almond butter, or
small protein shake

## FOODS TO EAT DURING THIS PHASE
Drink plenty of fresh water (8-10 glasses), herbal teas, green tea
Eat as much cruciferous vegetables as you wish (according to food
sensitivities)
Grain foods from rice, millet, quinoa, buckwheat, tapioca
Fresh fruits, vegetables, beans, peas
Olive oil, flaxseed oil, coconut oil, all natural seasonings, sea salt
## FOODS TO AVOID DURING THIS PHASE
_**ALL ANIMAL PRODUCTS**_—**fish, turkey, chicken**
Any food that you know you are allergic
Dairy (milk, cheeses, yogurt, butter), eggs, margarine, shortening
Foods prepared with Gluten-containing cereals like wheat, oats,
rye, barley, those ingredients normally found in breads, pasta, etc.
Tomatoes and tomato sauces, corn, peanuts
Alcohol, caffeine (coffee, black tea, soda), sweeteners
Soy products, beef, pork, conventional cold cuts (Oscar Mayer),
bacon, hotdogs, canned meat, sausage, shellfish, meat substitutes
Fried Food, dried fruit, fruit juice

**\*\*\*\*\*\*(NOTICE PROTEIN IS RE-INTRODUCED)\*\*\*\*\*\***
**COMPLETION PHASE 3 - SAMPLE MENU - _DAYS 15 TO 17_**

| | |
|---|---|
| **Breakfast** | Protein Shake, 1 serving before breakfast<br>1 serving: *Turkey* or *Chicken*<br>or<br>1 serving: Steel Cut Oatmeal or Gluten Free rolled oats (may use 1 packet of Stevia to sweeten)<br>and 1 serving: Fresh Fruit (Stick with berries or pitted fruit) |
| **Morning Snack** | (Not mandatory) Nuts, *animal protein* or *protein* supplement shake |
| **Lunch** | Green or spinach salad with *chicken breast*/ Olive Oil dressing<br>Steamed/ raw/grilled/baked vegetables |
| **Afternoon Snack** | (Not mandatory) Nuts, *animal protein* or *protein* supplement shake<br><br>Protein Shake 1 serving before dinner |
| **Dinner** | 1 serving: *Fish* or *Chicken breast* or *Turkey*<br>Brown rice & Steamed/ raw/grilled/baked vegetables or beans/peas<br>Green salad |
| **Nighttime Snack** | (Not mandatory) vegetable, almond butter or<br><br>small protein shake |

## FOODS TO EAT DURING THIS PHASE

Drink plenty of fresh water (8-10 glasses), herbal teas, green tea
Eat as much cruciferous vegetables as you wish
Grain foods from rice, millet, quinoa, buckwheat, tapioca
Fresh fruits, vegetables, beans, peas

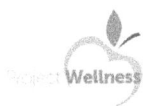

Fish, chicken, turkey *if* cold cuts-> (Organic /**no**
additives/nitrates/nitrites/growth hormones/MSG/preservatives
USDA Certified organic is best or Farmer's Market Produce)
Olive oil, flaxseed oil, coconut oil, all natural seasonings, sea salt

## FOODS TO AVOID DURING THIS PHASE

Any food that you know you are allergic
Dairy (milk, cheeses, yogurt, butter), eggs, margarine, shortening
Foods prepared with Gluten-containing cereals like wheat, oats,
rye, barley, those ingredients normally found in breads, pasta, etc.
Tomatoes and tomato sauces, corn, peanuts
Alcohol, caffeine (coffee, black tea, soda), sweeteners
Soy products, beef, pork, conventional cold cuts (Oscar Mayer),
bacon, hotdogs, canned meat, sausage, shellfish, meat substitutes
Fried food, dried fruit, or fruit juices

## COMPLETION PHASE 4 - SAMPLE MENU - *DAYS 18 TO 21*

**Breakfast**

Protein shake, 1 serving before breakfast
1 serving: Turkey or Chicken
OR
1 serving: Steel Cut Oatmeal Gluten Free rolled
oats (may use 1 packet of Stevia to sweeten)
AND 1 serving: Fresh Fruit (Stick with berries or
pitted fruit)

**Morning Snack**

(Not mandatory) Nuts, animal protein, or protein
supplement shake

**Lunch**

Fresh green/spinach salad with Olive Oil dressing
Steamed/raw/grilled/baked vegetables
Fish–broiled or baked

**Afternoon Snack**

(Not mandatory) Nuts, animal protein, or protein
supplement shake

**Dinner**

1 serving: Turkey or Chicken Breast or Fish–
broiled or baked

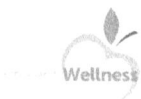
Steamed/raw/grilled/baked vegetables, beans or peas, salad

**Nighttime Snack**     (Not mandatory) vegetable, almond butter, or small protein shake

## FOODS TO EAT DURING THIS PHASE

Drink plenty of fresh water (8-10 glasses), herbal teas, green tea
Eat as much cruciferous vegetables as you wish
Grain foods from rice, millet, quinoa, buckwheat, tapioca
Fresh fruits, vegetables, beans, peas
Fish, chicken, turkey
Olive oil, flaxseed oil, coconut oil, all natural seasonings, sea salt

## FOODS TO AVOID DURING THIS PHASE

Any food that you know you are allergic
Dairy (milk, cheeses, yogurt, butter), eggs, margarine, shortening
Foods prepared with Gluten-containing cereals like wheat, oats, rye, barley, those ingredients normally found in breads, pasta, etc.
Tomatoes and tomato sauces, corn, peanuts
Alcohol, caffeine (coffee, black tea, soda), sweeteners
Soy products, beef, pork, conventional cold cuts (Oscar Mayer), bacon, hotdogs, canned meat, sausage, shellfish, meat substitutes, shellfish
Fried food, dried fruit, or fruit juices

Congratulations, AGAIN! Now that you have reached this point, you have accomplished some major victories in regaining your health and vitality. You have completed Phase 1 and 2. You may not realize it, but you have:

1) Eliminated common food sensitivities that may up-regulate the neuroendocrine-immune axis and lead to dis-ease;
2) Detoxified your system of accumulated toxins, heavy metals, metabolic debris, sludge & waste products;
3) Established a more functional environment for body systems;

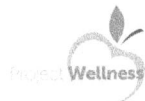

4) Cleared pathways for better digestion, filtration, elimination, & receptor activity;
5) Prepared your body for better metabolism, weight management, & nutritional utilization.

Now you can begin to add (1's and 2's on your food sensitivity list) foods back into the diet one at a time. For the next month, keep a dietary journal (the 24 Hour Daily Nutrition Summary) of what you eat including meals, snacks, and beverages. Use the food guide or go to www.calorieking.com or www.myfitnesspal.com to calculate your caloric intake. It is very important to "feed" your body good whole nutrient dense foods on a consistent basis (3-4x/day). Your body needs the appropriate caloric intake on a daily basis for your metabolism to work to optimum levels. You should now know that weight loss is not as simple as calories in-calories out. Many patients actually don't eat enough. By keeping this log, we can ensure you are getting what your body needs. Bring the logs in for doctor review each week. Also record how you feel with the food that was eaten. Keep a record of your daily exercise routine. You can use the exercise logs in the Project Wellness Workbook.

If supplementation is prescribed, it is for a specific reason. Be sure to follow the prescribed regimen. Additionally, a daily dose of protein supplement with repair enzymes and anti-inflammatories may be beneficial to your program and overall health. Drink one serving of vegetable protein drink just before breakfast, or as a mid-morning snack.

Remember, you now have a daily nutritional and exercise program and a care plan to provide your body with optimum nutrition, function, repair, recovery, and wellness. This is part of your lifestyle now. Eat according to the plan laid out for you. Drink plenty of fresh water. Include nutritionally rich foods. Love and care for your body and it will respond the way you want. You have already come a long way and laid the foundation to the new YOU. Great job! Let's keep your progress going full steam ahead. If you have any questions, ask! Remember, we are a team and we are in this together for the entire journey to wellness.

Pat yourself on your back! You did it!

Wellness

# Understanding Supplements

## Vitamins and minerals

Supplements are what we take to get the vitamins, minerals, antioxidants and nutritional needs met that we are unable to meet through what we eat or to combat the bombardment of artificial substances, toxins and environmental insults that we incur every day.

Vitamins and minerals are the most important part of health. What is a vitamin? What is a supplement? Do you need to take supplements?

Vitamins are organic compounds essential for growth, development and metabolism. Many cannot be synthesized by our body and must be supplied through diet or gastrointestinal intake. Vitamins and minerals come from plants and the soil. Lack of vitamins creates every known symptom and disease that you can describe. Being able to absorb essential nutrients is the key. Whether you get it from organic food supply in adequate amounts or take it in supplement form you still have to be able to absorb them so you must have a healthy gastrointestinal tract first.

Vitamins are not fuel or sources of energy. But they are the "ignition switch" used to turn on the engine. They are used as co-factors to form enzymes (biologic catalysts) that perform every process in your body or metabolism.

If you have a symptom or abnormality in your health, no matter what it is, it is a vitamin or mineral deficiency. The key is to know which one and then make sure that you can absorb it, use it and process it optimally.

Supplements are vitamins or minerals that you take other than whole food sources. Plant based supplements are called "Neutriceuticals".

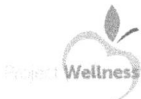

Quality really does matter with supplements and the process is critical to the effectiveness and the body's ability to absorb and process them.

You may ask, "Do I really need to take supplements?"

Many patients have told me that doctors tell them as long as you eat pretty healthy you don't need to take vitamins. Well first of all they are talking about supplements and second of all WHO REALLY EATS PRETTY HEALTHY??? I am the healthiest eater that I know and I struggle to get 10-12 servings of vegetables a day without juicing or eating medical foods.

Our soil is mineral depleted because farmers rarely turn over the crops as they should and is saturated with chemicals and pesticides that interfere with plant production of vitamins and minerals, so even if you ate tons of veggies you still wouldn't get what you need.

Even the United States Department of Agriculture has stated that over half of Americans are not getting the minimum RDAs (Recommended Dietary Allowances) through their current diet and this is with massive government fortification attempts.

Our food supply and intake has changed drastically over the past 40 years (I don't think anyone would dispute that) and as a result we are eating more chemicals, more processed foods and less nutrient dense foods packed with vitamins and minerals.

Doctors have been conditioned to treat with medications and many medications deplete precious vitamin stores through increased urinary excretion, blocking absorption, binding to nutrients and deactivating them, reducing stomach acid which begins the process of absorption, and increased loss through liver, kidneys and stool.

What's worse is that mediations kill more than 100,000 people in the U.S. every year according to JAMA and the CDC and this is as

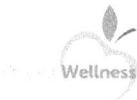

prescribed! That's more in a year than people died in the whole Vietnam War. There are over 10 million adverse reactions to FDA approved drugs a year. Vitamins kill no one and without them we are disease waiting to happen.

If you want to preserve your life and health you must supplement. You don't have to go crazy and spend huge amounts of money but you do need a road map to help you choose your supplements in the most wise and health efficient manner.

Symptoms are easy to go by and choose supplements to rectify, but the problem with that is that by the time you have symptoms you are so depleted that it may take what we call mega doses to return the body to health and wellness.

Take iodine for example. In the U.S. we began seeing children with large thyroid goiters from iodine deficiency. When the government and scientists convened and decided to fortify the foods with iodine, only amounts were added that would prevent goiter. Not optimal levels that would go beyond disease. And you know where they put it… In the salt. Which was a good bet because everybody eats salt so they are sure to get the iodine but it's not optimal levels. And what if you are avoiding salt? Which even people, who say they don't use salt, are probably not aware that they are getting massive amounts in processed foods and eating out.

Folic acid is another catastrophic misstep in my opinion. The government realized that we weren't getting enough folate (B9 vitamin that comes from foliage or green leafy vegetables thus the word folate) and we started having issues with Spina Bifida and neural tube birth defects. The scientists said, "folic acid is the same thing", but it wasn't. Just like the commercial where the mom picks up her son from school and he says, "your not my mom" and she says,

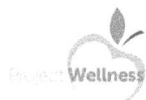

"Well, I'm age range 30-40, blond hair and drive a SUV… Close enough…" but it's not close enough and if you can't process or methylate folic acid, it accumulates as homocysteine and increases your risk of heart disease, stroke, infertility, cancer…. Etc. and so some supplements are not close enough but actually detrimental. You must take adequate amounts of methyl-folate to get optimal results.

B12 is interesting as well. We often use a cheap form that has a long shelf life called cyano-cobalamin. The cyan portion is actually cyanide molecule. Now you can argue that a little cyanide is not dangerous or that a little arsenic or mercury is not dangerous but I would argue that. It cost's more to by methyl-B12 instead of cyano-B12 and it costs more to buy good quality fish oil or omega-3 that don't have mercury contaminant but the difference is your health and your life. Empower yourself to know the score!

Essential Vitamins are broken down into water soluble and fat-soluble. The difference is that water soluble are easily excreted through the body if not needed or in excess and fat soluble may accumulate in the fat or adipose tissue and may accumulate in excess amounts, competing for other vitamins if not balanced.

**Water-soluble Vitamins**
B-vitamins
Vitamin $B_1$ (thiamine)
Vitamin $B_2$ (riboflavin)
Vitamin $B_3$ (niacin or nicotinic acid)
Vitamin $B_5$ (pantothenic acid)
Vitamin $B_6$ (pyridoxine, pyridoxal, pyridoxamine)
Vitamin $B_7$ (biotin)
Vitamin $B_9$ (folate)
Vitamin $B_{12}$ (cobalamine)
Choline and Inositol

Vitamin C (ascorbic acid)

**Fat Soluble Vitamins**
Vitamin A
Vitamin D
Vitamin E
Vitamin K

Minerals are different than vitamins. Minerals are also important to the production of enzymes and therefore essential for hormone production. Minerals also help the tissues and blood from becoming too acidic or too alkaline. Most people struggle with too much acidity, which can cause tissues to break down and predispose to disease. Some minerals like sodium, potassium and calcium have electrical charges that conduct electrical impulses along nerves and control muscle, brain and heart function. These minerals regulate fluid and also bind to protein and other organic substances, cell membranes and enzymes and act as catalysts for all body processes.

Essential minerals also called macro-nutrients because they are needed in large amounts include
-calcium
-potassium
-phosphorous
-sulfur
-sodium
-chloride
-magnesium
and micronutrients (needed in smaller amounts) include
-iron
-zinc
-selenium
-manganese
-copper
-cobalt
-iodine
-molybdenum

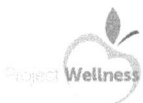

-chromium
-boron
-vanadium

Possibly Detrimental minerals that may compete for macro or micronutrients
-arsenic
-barium
-bromine
-cadmium
-germanium
-selenium
-tin
-nickel
-bismuth

Factors that can cause vitamin or mineral depletion:
Tobacco
Sugar
Antibiotics
Surgery
Diuretics
Fluoride
Pollution
Extreme heat or cold
Hormone imbalance (namely cortisol and estrogens)
Rancid fats
Medications such as aspirin, tranquilizers, laxatives, sleeping pills, birth control, antacids, ibuprofen, naproxen, diet pills, allergy pills and countless other medications
Illness
Pesticides
Pregnancy
Lactation
Salt
Emotional stress

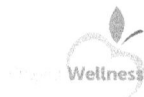

Mineral oil
Accidents
Food additives
Chlorinated or fluorinated water
Unhealthy diet
Soda Pop....
And the list goes on and on.

Herbs are valuable sources of natural medicine and have curative effects by balancing the vitamins and minerals and possibly any competing properties that toxins or adverse minerals or unbalanced proportions may have on our system.  Every plant on earth has some potential to help us symbiotically balance whatever may be going on with us.  We were meant to consume plants to provide us everything that we need.  Herbs contain powerful pharmaceutical agents.  About a third of all our medications or drugs are derived from a plant base.  The problem is that some of the pharmaceutical companies have changed the molecular structures in order to patent medications, which the body often cannot assimilate or recognize for intended natural processes.  The same thing happened with synthetic hormones.  You cannot patent something that God made, so you have to change it in some way.  These changes can cause a whole host of issues.

Many herbs cannot only treat symptoms and disease but may be used preventatively.  When used with good nutrition, exercise, adequate sleep and stress reduction can be a powerful adjunct to override genetic issues when the body is stressed.

Anti-oxidants are very important to health and wellbeing.  Everyday we are bombarded with chemicals and unnatural toxic exposures.  Our immune systems often cannot tolerate the toxic loads and damage is done to our cells.  I had a professor say one time, "look around the room… everyone in here has cancer….it's how the immune system handles it and repairs the DNA that either allows or permits dangerous or life threating tumor growth or bulk to form."

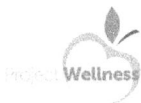

Wow! We all have cancer. It's true and we have to keep our immune system healthy to fight renegade life ending processes. That's not to scare us but to make us aware that we must protect the delicate balance.

My father died of cancer when I was nineteen. He worked as a TV repairman for many years and he often told me that the ionizing radiation from the TV tubes would probably some day cause cancer in him. He also understood the microwave radiation and dangerous environmental factors could create disease and cancer. He was right. I will never forget his words and strive everyday to keep my environment as clean as possible given the technology and chemicals in today's world. We can't control everything we are exposed to and I'm not likely to give up my computer or cell phone, but I can do everything in my power to combat the free radical effect in my cells. That's where anti-oxidants come into play.

What is a free radical? It is a molecule that has lost a vital piece of itself or one of its electrically charged electrons that normally orbit in pairs. To restore balance, the free radical steals electrons from nearby molecules or tries to give away its unpaired piece. This wreaks havoc in the DNA and can disfigure or corrode it. Causes damage and ultimately proteins, which make hormones to be produced that are defective.

If the free radical hits a protein it can destroy a cells ability to function. If it hits the DNA it can cause disease and cancer or stress the coding process. Aging is a direct effect of this renegade dangerous process. Ultimately we all die of the aging process.

It's sad when doctors tell patients who are ailing, "you are just getting older...". What they should say is your free radicals are destroying your DNA coding process that makes all your proteins and hormones and better yet... here's how you repair it!"

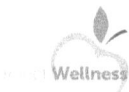

Anti-oxidant literally means against oxidation. They combat the effects of these free radicals. An antioxidant is a substance that can donate an electron to a free radical without becoming dangerous itself.

Anti-oxidants come in many forms. Ideally we want to get them from healthy plant foods.

The major anti-oxidants come from essential herbs, vitamins, minerals, amino acids, proteins and hormones and include
Vitamin A
Vitamin C
Vitamin E
Selenium
Beta Carotene
Bioflavonoids
Ginseng
Zinc
Molybdenum
Melatonin
Copper
Gingko Biloba
Pycnogenol
B-vitamins
N-Acetyl-Cysteine
Carotenoids (like lutein, zeaxanthin, lycopene…)
Garlic
Echinacea
Milk Thistle
CoQ10
ALA (Alpha-Lipoic Acid)
Glutathione
DHEA
Acetyl-L-Carnatine
CLA (Conjugated Linoleic Acid)

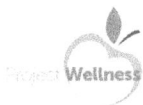

There is a big difference between pharmaceutical grade vitamins (medical grade) and their counterpart, store grade vitamins, or supplements. Now, this topic can get a bit fuzzy because it is very difficult to separate the need for a high-grade supplement and also realize that these supplements also need to be whole-food supplements.

These are two different topics but you must remember that just because a supplement is pharmaceutical grade does not mean it will be absorbed as well as one that is pharmaceutical grade that is not whole-food based, chelated, or attached in a way to add to the absorbability of the supplement. On the other hand, just because a supplement is derived from concentrated forms of whole food does not necessarily mean that it is what it says!

There are basically three major types of grades pertaining to what is in a product. Of course, the lowest on this scale would be that of feed grade, which is suitable for animal consumption. We won't even talk about that one! The middle classification is food grade, which many call store grade, and the last is pharmaceutical grade or what some term, medical grade. When we are talking about supplements, let's begin the discussion of food grade vitamin supplements. What are they? Simply put, food grade supplements can allow capsules that include only 20% of what they say they contain. They may contain all of the ingredients in a batch but not per capsule, so you really don't know what you are taking.

Have you ever read articles citing the incidence of "Port 'o Potty" companies finding hundreds of dissolved vitamins at the bottom of the screen filter? This happens because many vitamin supplements are not absorbed at all. They are so poorly absorbed, in fact, that the brand name can still be read on the tablet found on this filter. This is caused by the lack of bioavailability found in food-grade vitamins.

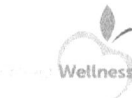

So the two major factors in using pharmaceutical grade vitamins would be one of bioavailability and the other . . . that you might want to know what you are ingesting!

In short, pharmaceutical grade supplements must meet the USP, or the United States Pharmacopeia standards. The USP provides assurance to consumers of the purity of the capsule. It must contain in excess of 99% of the ingredients stated. In addition to this, the bioavailability is much higher in pharmaceutical based supplements than that of store or food grade vitamins.

You need to ensure the bioavailability of supplements into your system, or you are wasting your money and worst of all the benefits of supplementing and working towards a good quality of life.

Choosing a vitamin or nutrient supplement is going to be imperative for your life today and into the future. Choosing one with phytonutrients, one that includes ingredients that reduce inflammation and help detoxify the liver, and one that includes micro nutrients such as vitamins and chelated minerals, will help you maintain your health.

We use many supplements in our office and through my years of research find that it is imperative that you only take medical grade or pharmaceutical grade supplements. We use only a few companies and much deliberation is put into the individualization of directing the use.

First and foremost we use supplements to heal the digestive tract, because until you do that you cannot absorb even the best supplements or extract nutrients from the food you consume.

Healing the gut usually starts with the following protocol:
Step 1: Betaine HCL to restore healthy hydrochloric acid balance to better digest the supplements

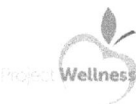

Step 2: Digestive enzymes and liver detoxification (B-vitamins, specifically methyl folate) with gall bladder support
Step 3: Anti-inflammatories, anti-oxidants and amino acids that repair and restore the delicate digestive lining
Step 4: Pro-biotics to restore the normal healthy intestinal flora
Step 5: Immune boosting vitamins like Vitamin D, and Vitamin C
Step 6: Minerals like magnesium to aid in intestinal motility
Step 7: Adrenal, thyroid and ovarian/testicular support to aid in overall absorption

With these steps covered then you can do individualized lab testing to identify areas that are deficient based on symptoms like fatigue, brain fog, autoimmune, allergies, joint pain, etc. At the least a B12, iron and Vitamin D level should be obtained as well as food allergy/sensitivity testing.

A good practitioner will guide you in supplements to cover deficiencies and amounts. It is very important that you work with someone who is knowledgeable about using supplementation to optimize health.

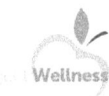

# Project Exercise

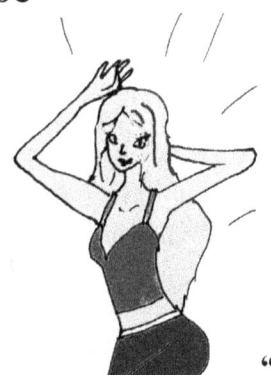

"

Okay. This doesn't have to be hard. Yay!

11 minutes a day? Do you have 11 minutes a day? Here's my simple plan to get you in shape.

(First, make sure that you are healthy enough to exercise by getting a physical medical examination from your doctor.)

1. Put on some really fast music and get a timer.

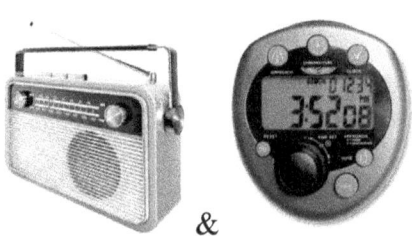

&

   5.   Stretch lightly for 30 seconds
   6.   Do the following exercises for 11 minutes in intervals.

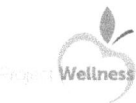
20 seconds run in place as HARD as you can
20 seconds rest

20 seconds punch in the air as hard as you can
20 seconds rest

20 seconds get up and down from a chair as fast as you can
20 seconds rest

Repeat circuit x 5 then 1 minute cool down/stretch
Or do a combination of the following exercises in 20 minute cycles as above.
Mix and match to avoid getting bored.

Journal what exercises you do each day to keep track and introduce variety.

OPTIONS:

Exercise Ball:  Sit ups and crunches

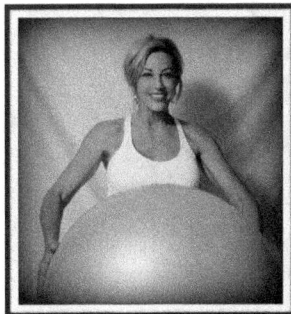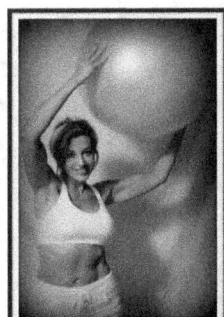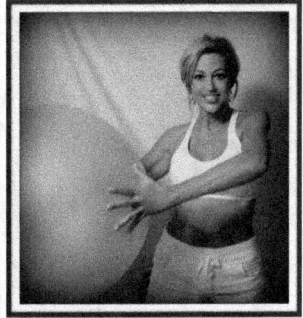

**Exercise Ball: Round the world**
Start with your exercise ball above your head, arms extended, then rotate the ball clockwise for 5 reps then counterclockwise for 5 reps. A stay ball with sand in it really works your arms.  Suck in your abs while you do this exercise for more abdominal work.

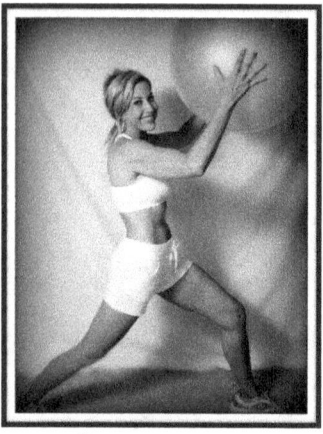

Lunges

Stand with ball in front of you and lunge forward then pull the ball into your extended knee and repeat 11 reps.

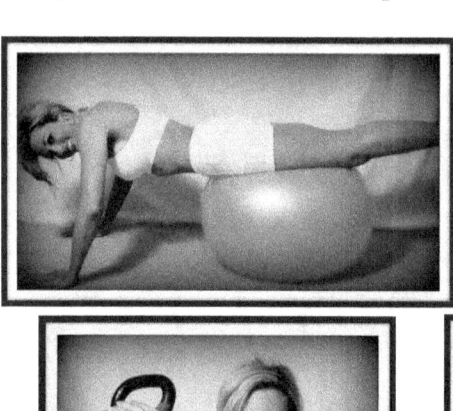

Push-ups

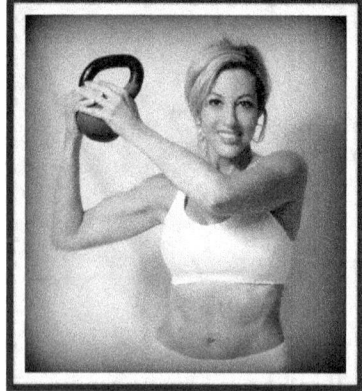

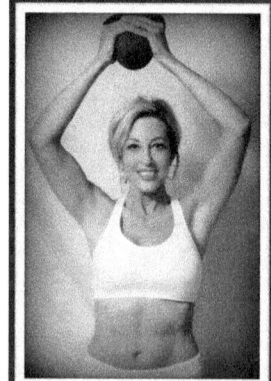

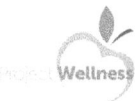

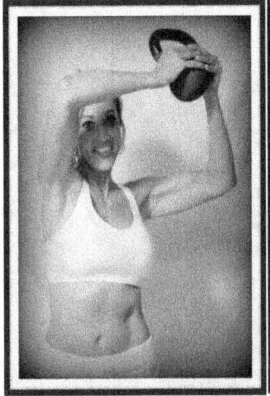 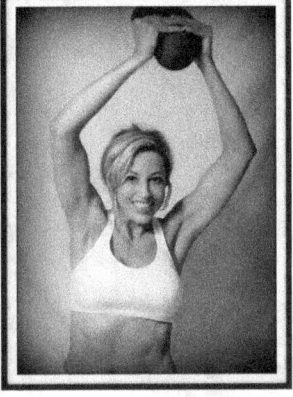

**Kettle Bell: Round the world**

Same things as with the ball but now with a heavier weight. Start
with 3lb. kettle bell. Never lift more than you can handle with
muscle fatigue.

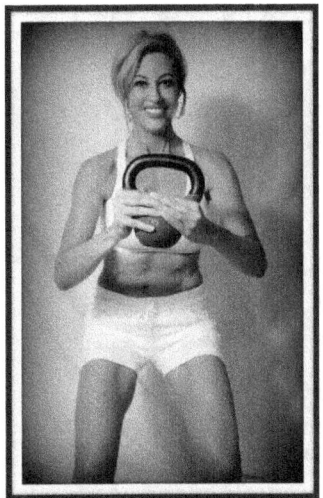 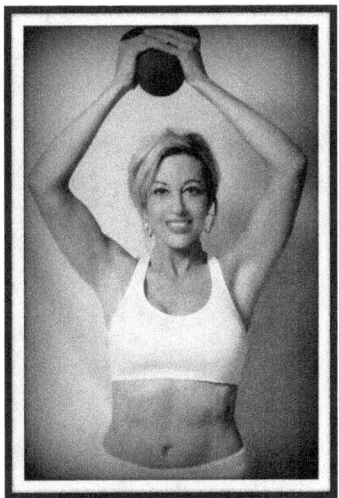

**Ski bumps**

Hold kettle bell in front and
bend knees, like you are going
Over little bumps skiing.

**Hula-hoop**

Hold kettle bell overhead
and rotate hips like you
are doing a hula-hoop.

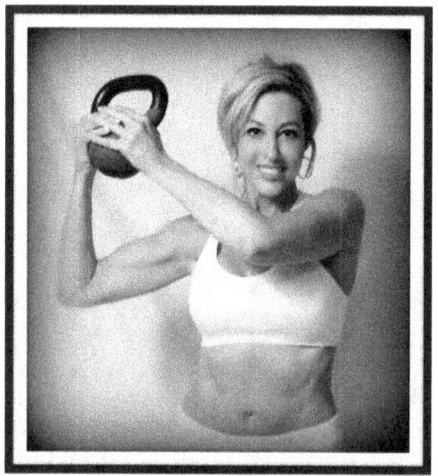

**Throws**
Kettle bell up over shoulder and
drop down to opposite knee.
Drops

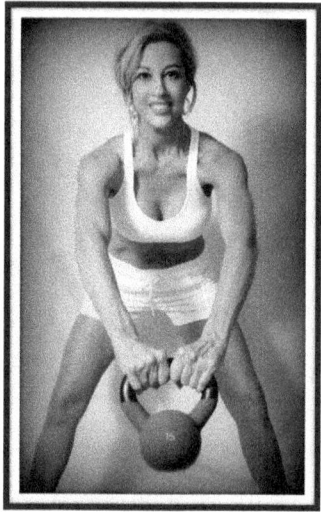

**Drops**
Kettle bell throws into
the middle of the inner
thighs and back out.

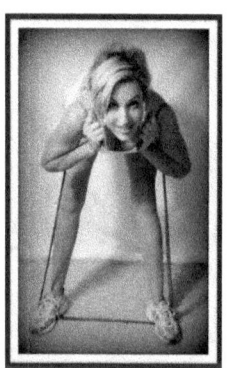

**Band: Froggies**

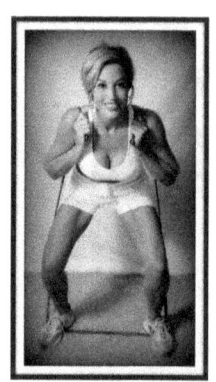

**Band: Squats**

Bend over with the Band around your
Shoulders and feet.  Keep your abs
Vertical with the floor and bend your
Knees.  11 rep

Squat all the way down
to your knees buttocks to
ankles.  11 reps

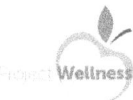

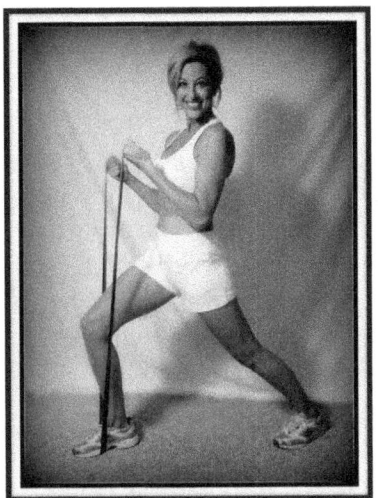

**Band: Lunges**
Band stretched out, lunge
deep bending back leg.
bends.  11 reps

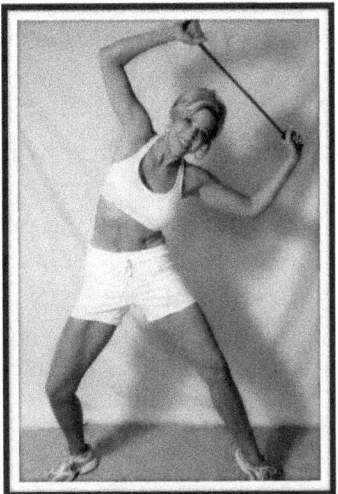

**Band: Side Bends**
Use band to stretch side
side  to  side  overhead.
 11 reps

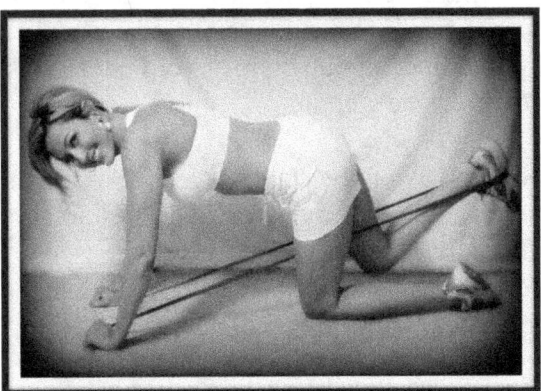

**Band: Donkey Kicks**
Stretch band behind and kick out
behind.  11 reps

TIPS: Don't eat within 1-2 hours of your workout or you will just burn the calories you consumed, defeating your purpose.  You want to burn the "stored stuff."  You want your insulin level low and keep it low during the workout.  You can drink all the water you want.   Watch the sports drinks as they usually have lots of carbs.

Exercise is effective in slowing aging and in helping to prevent heart disease, arthritis, osteoporosis, and other diseases of aging.  It also strengthens bones and muscles.  Exercise prevents arthritis, most likely, because a well-conditioned muscular system keeps the body in proper alignment. Since muscles hold the skeletal system in place, weak and out-of-shape muscles cause the body to be poorly aligned anatomically. When joints become crowded, their natural gaps and lubrication is reduced, so grinding during movement wears them down even further.

You must be careful not to "over exercise" because if you push beyond your metabolic capabilities you become subject to a variety of ailments including tissue damage hormone imbalance immune system dysfunction or injury.  Combined with the use of performance-enhancing drugs, such as anabolic steroids and amphetamines, many athletes are destroying their health in their quest for glory. Exercise must be part of a healthy lifestyle, including a good diet and nutrition.  Avoid negative habits, like smoking and excessive alcohol.

Exercise does not have to be stereotypical or extremely difficult but good exercise should provide extra demand on your system that is not normally experienced.  Many patients say "Well, I walk all day at work."   As I said earlier, with extra demands (not normal experiences) your body will adapt to the new (good) stress and become conditioned, stronger and healthier.  This means you should change your exercise routines regularly as well.

You must exercise correctly and learn how to do it without causing injury.  You need to educate yourself and also know your goals.  If you perform below your expectations on some days, it is ok.  Your

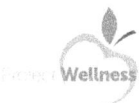

body has its own biorhythms and will fluctuate in energy and strength from one day to another.

The biggest thing is to do something you enjoy and just do it.

Remember you're never too old to start exercising. Start now! It doesn't matter how old you are. Exercise can also slow down cognitive or mental decline changes that often accompany aging. Exercise has also been shown to increase learning and memory by doubling the number of cells in a part of the brain called the hippocampus. Exercise has been shown to improve immunity, reduce body fat, and improve mood states. It is a known fact: regular exercise improves glucose metabolism and insulin sensitivity and reduces cholesterol levels.

While exercise is wonderful, there are circumstances when it can do more harm than good. Over-exercising or incorrectly exercising is stressful on the joints and can cause something called oxidative stress. Those who eat poorly, smoke, or do drugs can really increase the risk of oxidative stress while exercising. If you live in areas of high ozone, oxidative stress can be worsened. Taking supplemental antioxidants can reduce this oxidative stress.

You have to move it and love it! Always remember… challenge equals change! You constantly have to challenge yourself to improve your body contour, tolerance levels and fat burning qualities.

A word about Yoga. "He's in the zone!"
Sports fan or not, there's a pretty good chance that you're familiar with this expression.

"The Zone" is that special place where an athlete is locked in, so to speak. If you've played sports, you may have had your moments in it, but we tend to recognize and remember those who do it on the biggest of stages. It's like the night Reggie Jackson hit 3 home

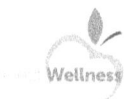
runs in the World Series on 3 consecutive pitches, or when
Michael Jordan dropped 63 on the Celtics in the playoffs. You can
feel that they're in a different place. It's as if they know they're
experiencing rarefied air, and they know that they're going to be
successful. You might hear an announcer suggest that they must be
"unconscious," when in actuality; the truth is that they are fully
conscious, just on another level!

You don't have to play professionally to know what it is to be in
the zone. In baseball, the ball looks like a beach ball coming to the
plate. In basketball, you get a rhythm going so sweet that you can
almost see the ball swishing through the net before it ever leaves
your fingertips, And in golf, you feel like you could take every
swing blindfolded. That is the zone. Every sport has that potential
experience. You see plays happening before they do. You are fully
present. Confident. Fearless. Grounded.

There is an inner calm, but intense focus at the same time. The
zone is simply a state of being.

Most amateur athletes have probably experienced it by way of
initial success breeding confidence and then a sudden recognition
of "being on a roll," basically. The goal may then become to hang
onto it instead of just being "in it," which actually causes it to fade.
States of being can be accessed, experienced and felt, but not
forced. In fact, it is the act of letting go that enables us to maintain
the experience itself – letting go of the results. THAT is true
fearlessness. You already know.

Frankly, a regular yoga and meditation practice teaches us how to
access this exact state of being. We are dipping into a sense of
"inner knowing" giving us the ability to see the present moment
for all that it is, and to let go of all that it is not. For athletes this
might mean simply clearing the active, anxious mind and enabling
it to focus solely on the task at hand while allowing the body to do
what it has been trained to do thousands and thousands of times.

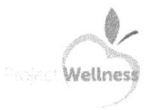

In other words, if we put our efforts into achieving inner calm, confidence and fearlessness, we can access the zone and put it into play in our competitive environments. I think most professional athletes will tell you that at a certain level, outside of those who are just incredibly superior physically and genetically gifted, what separates the super successful from the average guys is their mental approach to the game, and to their lives, I'm sure.

We love yoga in our wellness program. Here are some benefits of yoga.

1. Yoga improves your flexibility.
Improved flexibility is one of the first and most obvious benefits of yoga. During your first class, you probably won't be able to touch your toes, never mind do a backbend. But if you stick with it, you'll notice a gradual loosening, and eventually, seemingly impossible poses will become possible. You'll also probably notice that aches and pains start to disappear. That's no coincidence. Tight hips can strain the knee joint due to improper alignment of the thigh and shinbones. Tight hamstrings can lead to a flattening of the lumbar spine, which can cause back pain. And inflexibility in muscles and connective tissue, such as fascia and ligaments, can cause poor posture.

2. Yoga builds muscle strength.
Strong muscles do more than look good. They also protect us from conditions like arthritis and back pain, and help prevent falls in elderly people. And when you build strength through yoga, you balance it with flexibility. If you just went to the gym and lifted weights, you might build strength at the expense of flexibility.

3. Yoga prevents cartilage and joint breakdown.
Each time you practice yoga, you take your joints through their full range of motion. This can help prevent degenerative arthritis or mitigate disability by "squeezing and soaking" areas of cartilage

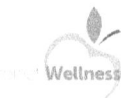
that normally aren't used. Joint cartilage is like a sponge; it receives fresh nutrients only when its fluid is squeezed out and a new supply can be soaked up. Without proper sustenance, neglected areas of cartilage can eventually wear out, exposing the underlying bone like worn-out brake pads.

4. Yoga builds better bone health and balance.
It's well documented that weight-bearing exercise strengthens bones and helps ward off osteoporosis. Many postures in yoga require that you lift your own weight. And some, like Downward- and Upward-Facing Dog, help strengthen the arm bones, which are particularly vulnerable to osteoporotic fractures. Also people who have decreased balance are more prone to falls and fractures. Regularly practicing yoga increases proprioception (the ability to feel what your body is doing and where it is in space) and improves balance. People with bad posture or dysfunctional movement patterns usually have poor proprioception, which has been linked to knee problems and back pain. Better balance could mean fewer falls. For the elderly, this translates into more independence and delayed admission to a nursing home or never entering one at all.

5. Yoga increases your blood flow.
Yoga gets your blood flowing. More specifically, the relaxation exercises you learn in yoga can help your circulation, especially in your hands and feet. Yoga also gets more oxygen to your cells, which function better as a result. Twisting poses are thought to wring out venous blood from internal organs and allow oxygenated blood to flow in once the twist is released.

6. Yoga drains your lymph system and boosts immunity.
When you contract and stretch muscles, move organs around, and come in and out of yoga postures, you increase the drainage of lymph (a viscous fluid rich in immune cells). This helps the lymphatic system fight infection, destroy cancerous cells, and dispose of the toxic waste products of cellular functioning.

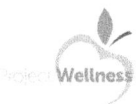

6. Aerobic Activity and ups your heart rate
When you regularly get your heart rate into the aerobic range, you lower your risk of heart attack and can relieve depression.

7. Yoga drops your blood pressure and regulates your adrenal glands.
Yoga lowers cortisol levels. If that doesn't sound like much, consider this. Normally, the adrenal glands secrete cortisol in response to an acute crisis, which temporarily boosts immune function. If your cortisol levels stay high even after the crisis, they can compromise the immune system. Temporary boosts of cortisol help with long-term memory, but chronically high levels undermine memory and may lead to permanent changes in the brain. Additionally, excessive cortisol has been linked with major depression, osteoporosis (it extracts calcium and other minerals from bones and interferes with the laying down of new bone), high blood pressure, and insulin resistance. In rats, high cortisol levels lead to what researchers call "food-seeking behavior" (the kind that drives you to eat when you're upset, angry, or stressed). The body takes those extra calories and distributes them as fat in the abdomen, contributing to weight gain and the risk of diabetes and heart attack.

8. Yoga lowers blood sugar.
Yoga lowers blood sugar and LDL ("bad") cholesterol and boosts HDL ("good") cholesterol. In people with diabetes, yoga has been found to lower blood sugar in several ways: by lowering cortisol and adrenaline levels, encouraging weight loss, and improving sensitivity to the effects of insulin. Get your blood sugar levels down, and you decrease your risk of diabetic complications such as heart attack, kidney failure, and blindness.

9. Yoga relaxes you.
Yoga encourages you to relax, slow your breath, and focus on the present, shifting the balance from the sympathetic nervous system

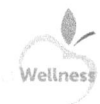
(or the fight-or-flight response) to the parasympathetic nervous system.

10. Yoga helps you sleep deeper.
Stimulation is good, but too much of it taxes the nervous system. Yoga can provide relief from the hustle and bustle of modern life.

11. Yoga prevents IBS and other digestive problems.
Yoga, like any physical exercise, can ease constipation—and theoretically lower the risk of colon cancer—because moving the body facilitates more rapid transport of food and waste products through the bowels. And, although it has not been studied scientifically, yogis suspect that twisting poses may be beneficial in getting waste to move through the system.

12. Yoga can keep you medication free.
If your medicine cabinet looks like a pharmacy, maybe it's time to try yoga. Studies of people with asthma, high blood pressure, Type II diabetes (formerly called adult-onset diabetes), and obsessive-compulsive disorder have shown that yoga helped them lower their dosage of medications and sometimes get off them entirely. The benefits of taking fewer drugs? You'll spend less money, and you're less likely to suffer side effects and risk dangerous drug interactions.

So if you didn't know why yoga was so amazing before, aren't these compelling reasons to at least try a class or two or more....

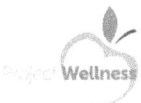

# Project Hormones

Hormones are the messengers of our bodies. They drive every process. When I say the word "hormone" everyone always thinks "estrogen" immediately and then the next thought is "estrogen causes cancer!" and they get completely shut down.

"I don't want any hormones." They say out of frustration or fear.

First of all you would die without hormones and second of all there are literally thousands of hormones swirling around in your body telling every cell what to do, when to do it, how to do it, etc. Even vitamin D is a hormone. You have sleep hormones, cholesterol hormones, metabolism hormones and every process in your body has hormones at the helm.

So how did I come to so intimately concern myself with hormones and how they work?

It all started with having every female problem that a girl can have from the time of about age nine. I had terrible pain and didn't start my periods until I was almost sixteen. They were heavy and terrible. They lasted weeks and consisted of needing super-plus tampons and having terrible cramps and PMS (pre-menstrual syndrome) symptoms. I was anemic and grumpy. Only later in life was I actually diagnosed with PCOS (polycystic ovarian syndrome) and endometriosis with huge fibroid tumors. I struggled with fertility for thirteen years because of these issues and had a miscarriage which was devastating. I was able to finally get pregnant but ended up with complications in the ICU at six months and almost died.

After my son was born I continued having terrible female issues and was diagnosed with the possibility of ovarian cancer. I underwent a hysterectomy and although it was not cancer this was just the beginning of a new set of female hormone issues. You see

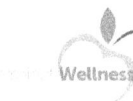

it didn't correct the underlying problem it just removed the organs that were being affected most by it.

I went on synthetic hormones and gained almost eighty pounds. I was miserable but at the time, even though I was a physician I didn't know that I had other options. They don't teach you about this stuff in medical school.

I am a doctor and I really had no clue how my own body really worked or how to fix it. Sure, I took biology and physiology, but no one ever told me what I really needed to know about hormones and the impact they have on the human body.

One day a patient came to my clinic, dressed professionally and quite eloquent with her words.

"Do you prescribe bio-identical hormones?" She asked, matter-of-factly.

"Bio what?" I asked.

"You know," she paused. "Natural hormone therapy… like Suzanne Somers uses."

I had no idea what she was talking about, so I looked at her more intently, leaned in, and said, "Tell me more."

She proceeded to tell me about natural hormone therapy and all the benefits of it. I was astounded. My jaw dropped as she told me about a world out there that was completely foreign to me. I thought hormone replacement therapy was bad, very bad. I thought it was only to be used for the woman who was soaking in sweat constantly or homicidal/suicidal.

I had received so much faulty information in medical school from pharmaceutical companies. They continue to feed us faulty

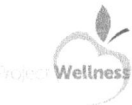

information.   Until that point, I believed a woman didn't need progesterone if she didn't have a uterus.  I was taught there was only one way to take hormone replacement therapy and only a couple of different options or doses.

I told my patient I knew nothing about what she was talking about, and I promised her I would find out.  I try to keep an open mind about alternative therapies.  Many physicians don't bother with alternative therapies because there is already so much to learn and know.  Why add more?  These physicians ask, "If there is no evidence-based research behind it (or at least that's what big pharmaceutical companies would have us believe), isn't it better to prescribe a pill?"  Some doctors cattle forty or more patients through their halls a day.  That doesn't leave much time to look into alternative therapies.  I feel very differently about this, and for this reason, I vowed to look into "bio-identical hormone therapy."

I did a Google search on Suzanne Somers and soon had unlocked a door to a world I never new existed.  That was six years ago.  So, what was the outcome?

Ms. T (me) started on bio-identical hormone therapy, and I prescribed it for that patient, too.  I lost over sixty pounds and escaped night sweats and hot flashes!  My mood was stable for once, and I was sleeping again.  I put testosterone in the prescription and actually got a libido back.  I felt better than I had felt since those nasty periods started when I was a teenager.

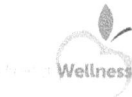

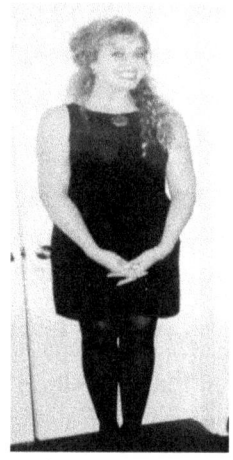
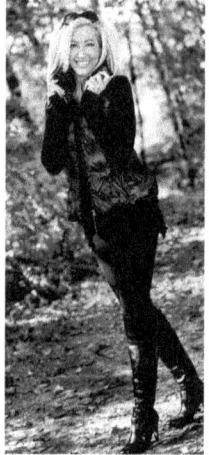

**Before: Age 37**       **After: Age 47**

I learned that my hysterectomy was probably not necessary. The abnormal pap, fibroids, and endometriosis found at the time of my surgery were all a product of my massive hormone imbalances. I learned my heavy periods were from the excess estrogen I was storing, when I unknowingly put on an extra ten pounds in college. From this and more, I have learned patients do not have to suffer and have unnecessary procedures and surgeries and rely on big pharmaceutical companies' answer to these issues.

So my journey began. I thank that woman every day for introducing me to something new. I didn't know it that day, but I had embarked on a journey. Looking back, this time was the beginning of "Project Fabulous," which has morphed into an overall wellness program called "Project Wellness."

So what are Hormones?

The word hormone comes from the Greek word *hormān* meaning to "urge on" or "impulse."

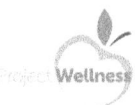

Hormones are more than just estrogen. When most people think about hormones, they think of estrogen and immediately fear comes to mind. Pharmaceutical companies have manipulated estrogen and made it unsafe, convinced doctors they have the only option, and created mistrust of "hormones." Amazingly, on a daily basis, patients tell me their doctor put them on estrogen after having a hysterectomy and told them they didn't need progesterone because they didn't have a uterus anymore. Let me explain why this is amazing to me.

Progesterone has so many more uses than just preventing lining buildup in the uterus. It's like saying that you don't need shoes because you're not wearing any socks, but as we all know, shoes have more functions than just covering up your socks. When patients tell me they are scared of hormones, I take a lot of time to undo the damage that big pharmaceutical companies have done. Their unnatural manipulation of the basic hormone structure given to women in unhealthy doses and distribution forms is not good.

We all have hormones. Some of my emphysema patients tell me they don't want to go on oxygen because they are afraid they will get addicted to it. HELLO?! We are ALL addicted to oxygen! We cannot live without it! Some people need a little purer form or an increased concentration of it to help the heart and lungs work more efficiently.

Pharmaceutical companies know hormones cannot be patented. God invented them. He has the ultimate patent. By the way, you can't patent oxygen either. For marketing purposes and sales, they figured out if they changed the structure, they could patent the new compound, and sell it for a lot of money. The problem is that the new compound is just different enough to cause problems. The amount is "one size fits all," and the route through the gastrointestinal tract and liver filtering creates inflammatory proteins causing all sorts of problems from joint aches to blood clots and, worse yet, cancer.

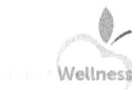
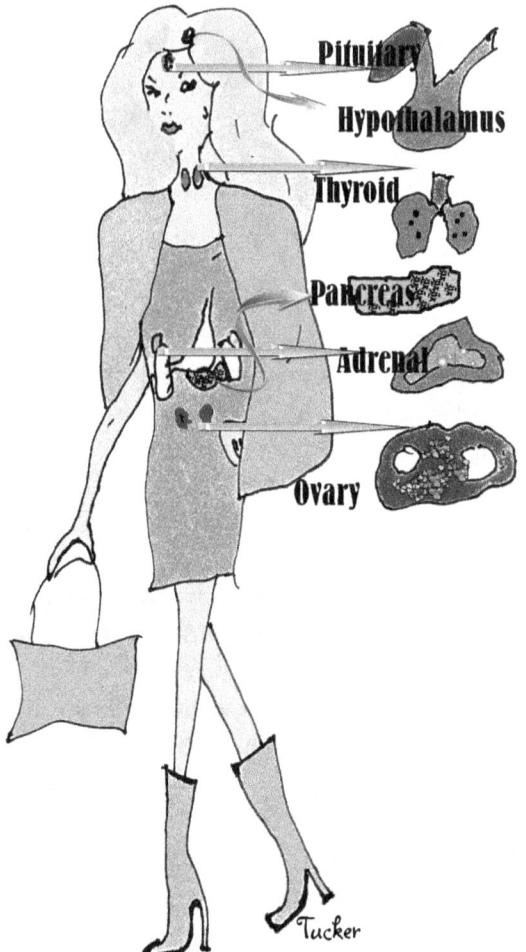

Remember, all hormones work in concert to balance each other. One is not more important than another. One may be more abundant at certain parts of the circadian rhythms, but they are always in balance.

Did you know you are a walking, talking, shopping bunch of hormones? Hormones control everything we are and do!

*Estrogen* – Makes us "girly"; induces puberty in females and facilitates the menstrual cycle in preparation for fertilization. Less known functions include libido, breast health, and enhancing female traits and characteristics.

*Progesterone* – Helps maintain menstrual cycle. It is more than just a hormone of uterine balance, however, because it helps with mood balance, sleep, and appetite or weight gain just to name a few of its purposes.

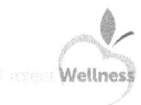

*FSH* – Causes menstrual cycle to START. This is a great marker as a blood test if you question whether or not you are in menopause. As the ovaries start to decompensate, FSH increases in the feedback loop. If your periods are irregular, this will help clarify menopause.

*LH* – Triggers ovulation and creates corpus luteum. In guys, it triggers production of testosterone.

*Insulin* – Comes from the pancreas and regulates sugar or carbohydrates in the blood stream. It does this by removing sugar from the blood stream, lowering the blood sugar level, and stores the glucose in various cells (usually fat). Therefore, when this hormone is elevated for long periods of time, it stops working effectively and you are likely to gain weight.

*Glucagon* – Is produced in the pancreas and functions to raise very low blood sugar. Glucagon is also used in diagnostic testing of the stomach and other digestive organs.

*Testosterone* – Makes guys look like "guys." It enhances and builds muscle (anabolic). It also maintains bone density, regulates hair growth, and maintains healthy libido or sexual interest. In males, it is primarily secreted from the testes, and YES, females have testosterone, too! It comes from the ovaries and sometimes from the adrenal glands. Males make about ten times as much as females, although females are more sensitive to its effects.

*Thyroxin* – Usually abbreviated as T4. Thyroxin is a prohormone meaning that it is inactive and must be converted to triiodothyronine (T3) or the active more potent form. It does this conversion in the target tissues and works to regulate just about every physiological process in the body, including, but not limited to growth, development, metabolism, body temperature, and heart

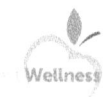

rate. It also helps as a lipid-modifying agent affecting weight gain and loss.

*TSH* – Is released from the pituitary gland in the brain and stimulates production of thyroid hormones. It is a very sensitive blood indicator for thyroid function.

*Aldosterone* – Comes from the adrenal gland and regulates sodium and potassium in the kidney. It increases blood pressure by retaining sodium. It may have further indications for hearing loss and ringing in the ears.

*Anti-diuretic Hormone* – Regulates water retention and blood pressure.

*Ghrelin* – produced mainly by the lining in the stomach and cells in the pancreas and stimulates hunger. It is considered the counterpart of the hormone leptin. Highly regulated by adequate sleep.

*Leptin* – (Greek *leptos* meaning thin) – which is made in fat cells and induces satiation when present at higher levels. Leptin plays a key role in regulating energy intake and energy expenditure, including appetite and metabolism.

*Melatonin* – "hormone of darkness" released from the pineal gland in the brain when the level of light is decreased and helps induce sleep. Closely balanced with leptin and ghrelin.

And these are just a few!

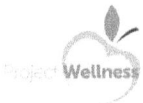

Understanding Yin and Yang.

The body is constantly trying to stay in balance. The hormones are intimately connected and in constant communication with each other. They are what Chinese philosophy calls "Yin and Yang." I believe that the universe itself is bound by balance and counterbalance. Yin and Yang encompasses the all-in-one belief that the earth and the universe, even, are all one system. There is no superiority, only balance. Each yields to the other without question. It takes a human mind to mess up the balance. Harmony is the balance of the system, and any deviation can drastically disturb it.

We live in a society where more is better. When we accept balance, we know this cannot be true. In every decision, there are pros and cons. This is the balance that the universe maintains over us. When we accept this concept, the body becomes an orchestra to be played with a conductor and we can understand how balance becomes the key issue. The concept of the universe and the moon and its lunar cycles ties us to something even bigger than ourselves; it's no coincidence that the moon takes approximately 28 days to orbit the earth and this about the time of a "normal" menstrual cycle. In fact, the same root word in Latin is *mensus* (to measure and menstrual) meaning month and echoes the moon's importance to measurements of time.

Also, of interesting note, every 223 months (also called a Saros cycle) the sun, moon, and moon's nodes align in the same relative angles to each other. This happens about every nine years. Then every 56 years, the elliptical position of the north node of the moon moves, and the sun's relative position will shift resulting in alternating solar/lunar eclipses. Is it coincidental that every nine years humans experience monumental changes? A nine-year-old child starts the hormonal changes that trigger puberty. An eighteen-year-old human starts the cycle of starting to establish societal roles. Thirty-six-year-old humans in our society are at the peak of child-rearing and at forty-five, many humans are experiencing their "mid-life crisis." Then in our fifties, we start the cycle of menopause (yes, men do, too), and then in our sixties, we start to experience significant age-related disease increases and become eligible for Medicare.

So, if we deny the Yin-Yang theory and fail to realize the balance of the universe, we may make many mistakes in our metabolic balance. Technologic advances have led the way to many ways we can counterbalance these lunar cycles. Pharmaceuticals now make chemicals (more on xenoestrogens and petrochemicals later) that interfere with our hormonal balances and ingest them on a daily basis.

Let me now describe a few patterns within the human body that clearly show the Yin-Yang balance.

Let's start with hormones. What comes to mind? Okay, probably estrogen. Well, if the Yin is estrogen, then the Yang would be progesterone. Progesterone's role in balancing estrogen is well established, and the feedback loop with one another is classic hormone science. What about insulin? If insulin is Yin, then, its Yang would be glucagon which has opposite effects but maintains the same goal of glucose metabolism and storage in body. While insulin lowers blood sugar, glucagon works to raise it.

What about the thyroid? Thyroid hormone balance (both active and inactive form) is achieved through feedback with TSH (thyroid stimulating hormone) from the brain.

Leptin and ghrelin are Yin-Yang hormones of hunger and satiety (fullness) and closely regulated by sleep.

Some hormones even have two names, like growth hormone balance. The Yang to growth hormone is the hormone

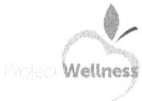

somatostatin and it is also called GHIH or growth hormone-inhibiting hormone. It also has the name, somatotropin release-inhibiting factor. That name alone establishes its Yin-Yang nature. Its unique properties are in its ability to regulate growth and also functions to regulate (feedback for inhibiting and releasing) many other hormones to stay in balance.

Some hormones are balanced also by the substrate or materials available within a closed system. For example, calcium concentration availability feeds back with a hormone called parathyroid hormone to keep calcium concentration balanced in the blood stream, but parathyroid hormone also has a Yang called calcitonin a hormone that lowers calcium levels in the blood.

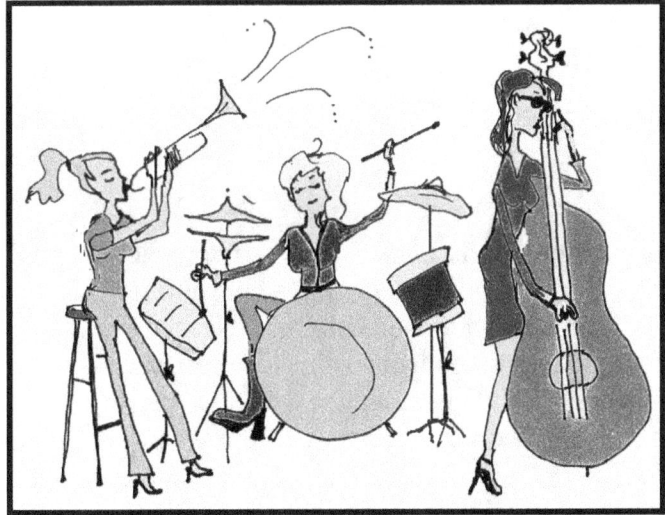

Like a fine tuned orchestra, every instrument has its own place and sound. When one is out of balance, all of the music sounds bad.

The biggest balancing act in the human body is the balance between the blood stream content and storage or usage of materials in the tissues. This balance is orchestrated starting with the HPA or hypothalamus/pituitary/adrenal axis.

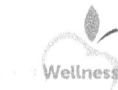
The HPA (hypothalamus-pituitary-adrenal) axis is no different and drives everything you do. Every thought. Every action. Hormones are all driven very intricately by a feedback loop intertwined with one another and delicately balancing the whole body.

The conductor, in this case, is "stress" and is responsible for deciding the players and the hormones roles with each other.

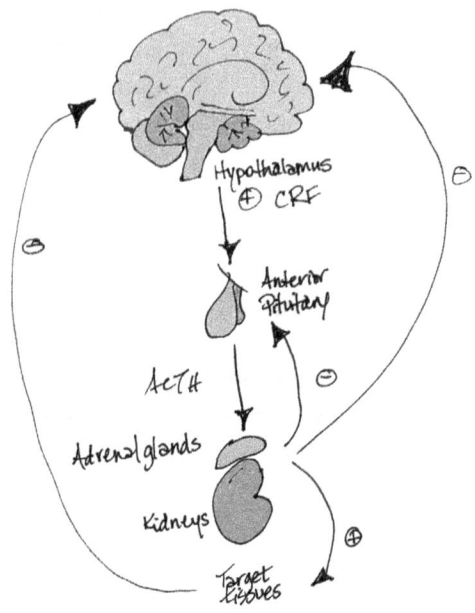

Important key and hormones do that. There are two major classes of hormones: PPA (protein, peptides, amino acids) and steroid hormones. PPAs bind to receptors on cells and alter the behavior of the cell. Sometimes opening channels into the cell and sometimes closing them or going straight to the nucleus (powerhouse of the cell) and turns genes off and on.

Steroid hormones go into cells and exert their power there, while PPAs work from the surface to trigger a cascade of events.

Did you know you actually need your cholesterol? All steroid hormones come from the cholesterol molecule. Since steroid hormones are made from cholesterol (or a fat molecule), it can easily slip into cell membranes that are fat-soluble. To keep them from just plopping into any cell, they usually catch a ride on "carrier proteins," like a "hormone taxi."

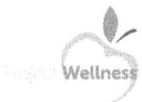

Steroid hormones are further grouped into five categories depending on what receptors they bind to. These are: glucocoricoids (sugar), mineralocorticoids (electrolyte balance), androgens (think testosterone), estrogens, and progesterones. Vitamin D is a close cousin to a steroid hormone.

A word about Insulin, the sugar storage hormone:

"But I'm not a diabetic!" You might be saying. Maybe you aren't and maybe you are. Maybe you are on your way to diabetes if you are not already there. I believe that everyone who is overweight is on their way to diabetes. It is a continuum of the mechanism of insulin to get sluggish and to eventually not work at all. Maybe you are on the front end. This is your chance to save yourself a lot of grief. If you have ever known a diabetic (and there's a good chance you do as nearly one in three Americans are), you know management of the disease is not much fun. There are needles, lots of needles. And giving up the foods you supposedly love? They are the very foods that got you in this mess.

The American Diabetes Association quotes the following statistics:

Under 20 years of age
- 215,000, or 0.26% of all people in this age group have diabetes
- About 1 in every 400 children and adolescents has type 1 diabetes

Age 20 years or older
- 25.6 million, or 11.3% of all people in this age group have diabetes

Age 65 years or older
- 10.9 million, or 26.9% of all people in this age group have diabetes

Men
- 13.0 million, or 11.8% of all men aged 20 years or older have diabetes

Women
- 12.6 million, or 10.8% of all women aged 20 years or older have diabetes

These are terrifying stats. I truly, personally believe this prevalence is due to high fructose corn syrup in our diets. The most abundant source is the SODA POP. A cute little bubbly drink that wakes us up and makes us feel good… is killing us. My biggest problem with the soda industry is that a soda is just a plain waste of calories. One of my mantras is "if it's not worth the calories…DON'T EAT IT!"

Did you know that an 8 oz. cola has 105 calories approximately. A 12 oz. can has 155 calories, a 16 oz. can has 200 calories, and a 22 oz. can has 280 calories!

Just to give you some perspective, there are about 200 calories in a small hot fudge sundae. I'd rather have the ice cream than the drink if I'm going to consume calories.

So that's it. Sodas are just empty calories. You are just as satisfied with water when your body adjusts to not having sodas anymore and you can save your calories for other things.

Of course, there are other more insidious reasons sodas are bad for you. They are straight carbohydrate. High fructose corn syrup was cultivated in our society because it was found to be a cheap source of sugar. The problem is that it is actually much worse for stimulating insulin production and causing weight gain. A study done by Princeton University showed high fructose corn syrup in rats with access to it were significantly fatter than those who had access to table sugar even though caloric intake was the same.

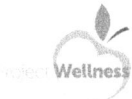
They found that it leads to long-term increases in body fat and raises triglycerides (sugary part of your cholesterol).

Studies show that high fructose corn syrup may be processed by the body differently. Fructose is metabolized to produce fat while glucose is processed as energy or stored as a carbohydrate in the muscles and liver. Researchers also point out that it is no coincidence that forty years ago approximately fifteen percent of the population was obese, now in 2011, thirty-three percent of Americans are obese.

Have you ever heard of a glucose tolerance test? If you are overweight and your doctor suspects that you may have diabetes, he or she may ask you to do a test called an oral glucose tolerance test, or OGTT. It measures your body's use of insulin and how effective it is at lowering the sugar content in the blood.

So, how is the test done? Well, you eat normally the week before the test. You shouldn't go crazy and should keep your carbs less than 150-200 grams of sugar/carbs day. Then you need to fast the night before the test (nothing at all for eight to twelve hours). A fasting blood sugar is then checked first thing when you arrive. If it is normal, then they give you a drink with 75 grams of carbohydrates. Then blood glucose levels are drawn at certain hourly intervals thereafter and monitored for abnormal elevations.

Okay, are you ready for this? This glucose drink is just a flat cola. No fizz and no fun. A twelve ounce can of soda has 39-55 grams of carbohydrates. So think of it this way. Every time you drink a couple of cans of cola you are giving your body a glucose tolerance test!

If we are testing how quickly glucose is metabolized from the bloodstream for use by cells as an energy source, and the normal rate of glucose clearing is impaired, and we keep challenging our

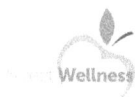

body in this way… well, common sense tells you THAT CAN'T BE GOOD!

Hopefully, I have convinced you to give up High Fructose Corn Syrup drinks whose carb grams are designed to make you gain weight. Water is sounding better by the second, right?

So, why do I tell you all this? My hope is you have a better appreciation of insulin and carbohydrates. Since this chapter is about insulin, let me explain a little more about how insulin works.

Our natural instincts as a human are to eat and store as much as you can. Our hormones are designed to work in our favor if you know how to maximize them, but they can work against you if you don't. If you do not control insulin, then it will control you. "Insulin? I'm not diabetic." You say to yourself, "What has insulin got to do with me?"

Insulin's function is quite simple in the body. It is to lower your blood sugar/glucose by moving it from the blood vessel to somewhere else for storage. That somewhere else unfortunately leads to being overweight.

Insulin (from the word *insula* in Latin, meaning "island") is a hormone that comes from an area in the pancreas called the islets (small island) of Langerhans. It is a peptide hormone that needs zinc to hold it together. Insulin is a powerful hormone constantly staying in balance with its yang twin glucagon.

Insulin is vital to regulation of carbohydrates and storage of fat. It is responsible for making liver, muscle, and fat tissue suck up carbohydrates. Carbohydrates can be many different kinds of sugars (glucose, fructose, lactose, etc.). From here on out, I will use the term sugar, glucose, and carbohydrate interchangeably. However, carbohydrates can be composed of many different sugars

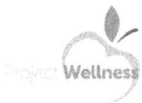

besides glucose.  When carbohydrates are out of the blood stream and stored in tissues, they become glycogen or stored sugar.

Insulin is in constant feedback with glucagon, the hormone that signals an increase in blood sugar.  If insulin has not been signaled to come out of its home, the pancreas, by elevated blood sugar levels then the body begins to use fat as an energy source for a process called gluconeogenisis that happens in the liver.  Another way of saying this is the fat cell's lipids (or mobile fat…again I might use fat or lipid interchangeably like the sugar/carbohydrate thing) go to the liver to form molecules of sugar.  Yes, the body can make its own sugar from materials present in storage.  This is why a diabetic can wake up with an elevated blood sugar in the morning even though they have not eaten in many hours through the night.  The liver gets extra busy.  An important fact to understand:  If you exercise on an empty stomach you are more likely to use up stored sugar than to burn the immediate source you just gave it (like a cookie).

Insulin does other things, like signal body tissues to take amino acids to make other hormones and it has anabolic, or growth effects on tissues as well.  It also influences blood vessel compliance (how narrow or big they become) and brain function or cognition, particularly spoken word memory.  Insulin also enhances learning.  It helps to regulate temperature in response to food intake which suggests that brain insulin levels contribute to control of total body energy expenditure.

When insulin no longer signals correctly, you will become diabetic.  As a consequence, you become insulin-deficient and eventually you may need to take insulin through a shot as a replacement.  This is usually a type 2 diabetic.  Type 1 diabetics cannot make insulin at all and possibly never could.

Insulin cycles in response to blood glucose levels.  There are usually three peaks during the course of twenty-four hours

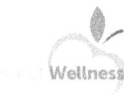

because, culturally, we eat three meals a day. Blood glucose may be low in the 70s when you wake up and spike up to 126 after a meal. Within a few hours, they both go back down if everything is working right and the cycle starts all over again. Ideally, if we ate five or six small carbohydrate loads/meals throughout the day, then we would never see a spike in glucose or resulting spike in insulin. The spikes and dips are responsible for overworking insulin as a hormone and making it work less effectively.

If insulin's role is to store sugar in the cells and get it out of the blood stream, then you are sure to gain some weight every time it surges. It's all about balance. This is also the reason that fasting does not work. When you do not eat for significant periods of time and your body is used to spiking and dipping, then you dip even lower with your blood glucose and the body regulates up to mobilize glucose accessibility. You are doing nothing to lose matter from the system, only rearranging it in an unstable way.

Why all this talk about insulin? As I mentioned before, anyone who is over weight is on a continuum to insulin resistance and eventually Type 2 diabetes.

Exercise (thirty to forty-five minutes, three to four times a week) can drastically increase your insulin sensitivity. Interestingly, when you exercise insulin levels decrease over time. If you haven't eaten a bunch of carbs before you exercise, your muscles use stored glucose since that is the only source.

This being said, if you consume a lot of carbohydrates right before you exercise, then the body will burn those and not the stored fat or carbs. You are defeating the purpose of exercise. If you exercise after having eaten, your insulin surges and your workout is essentially a bust. You only burn the calories you just consumed.

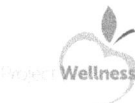

## Maximizing Your Sleep Hormones

Researchers say that how much you sleep and how well you sleep may silently orchestrate a symphony of hormonal activity tied to your appetite. According to the National Sleep Foundation, the average woman gets only six and a half hours of sleep per night. Chronic sleep deprivation can have a variety of effects on the metabolism and overall health.

You've heard it before. "Gotta get your beauty sleep." It's really true. If you don't get adequate sleep, you will have a very difficult time losing weight. The main reason is that when you don't get enough sleep a hormone called Ghrelin is released in excess. Ghrelin is a hormone that is known to stimulate appetite. Leptin is the yang of Ghrelin.

Leptin is known to decrease appetite and is abundant when sleep is adequate. Usually this is around 8-9 hours for the average adult. In 2006 at the American Thoracic Society International Conference, it was shown that women who slept 5 hours per night were 32% more likely to experience major weight gain (an increase of 33 pounds or more) and 15% more likely to become obese over the course of the 16-year study, compared to those who slept 7 hours a night. Those women who slept 6 hours per night were still 12% more likely to experience major weight gain and are 6% more likely to become obese, compared to women who slept 7 hours a night.

Just a few days of sleep restriction starts an abnormal cascade of hormone imbalances that increase hunger. Even if you eat less, you will still gain weight. Then, there is the impact of cortisol levels. When you don't get enough sleep, there is an increase in cortisol that also stimulates hunger, affects insulin, and may therefore add to unwanted weight gain. It does this by decreasing the ability to process carbohydrates, manage stress, and maintain a proper balance of hormones. In just one sleep-restricted week,

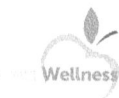
research study participants had a significant loss in their ability to process glucose and had an accompanying rise in insulin.

Your basal metabolic rate thermostat (calories you burn at rest) may be reset when you do not receive adequate sleep in a negative way. Also, those that don't rest well are tired and may not move around as much during the day to burn calories. Inadequate sleep can reduce levels of growth hormone that regulate the body's proportions of fat and muscle, so not only are you fat, but you'll be "lumpy."

As mentioned, sleep quality is important to assess as well. The hit show "The Biggest Loser" knows this, too. Since the show's seventh season, sleep studies have been added to the contestants' pre-show medical work-ups. Those with sleep apnea receive treatment. Doctors found that a majority of the contestants had sleep apnea. Unsurprisingly, a neck measurement of 17 inches puts you at great risk, and often severe cases. In one season, every cast member had a positive sleep apnea diagnosis according to the National Sleep Foundation's website. This website has an interesting interview of Sean Algaier and how sleep apnea affected his life.

The Greek word *apnea* literally means "without breath." There are three types of apnea: obstructive, central, and mixed. Of the three, obstructive is the most common. Despite the difference in the root cause of each type in all three, people with untreated sleep apnea stop breathing repeatedly during their sleep, sometimes hundreds of times during the night and often for a minute or longer.

Snoring is not normal. It runs the emotional gambit of cute to down right annoying to most. Marriages have ended over it. Some people think that it is okay to snore. It isn't. The sound of the snore is from a physical blockage of the airway or obstruction. Obstructive sleep apnea (OSA) is caused usually when the soft tissue in the rear of the throat collapses and closes during sleep. In

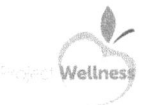 

central sleep apnea, the brain fails to signal the muscles to breathe. Mixed apnea, as the name implies, is a combination of the two. With each apnea event, the brain briefly arouses people with sleep apnea in order for them to resume breathing, but consequently sleep is extremely fragmented and of poor quality.

Sleep apnea is very common.

Risk factors include being male, overweight, and over the age of forty. It can affect anyone of any age, even kids. There seems to be an insurmountable lack of awareness by the public and healthcare professionals. The vast majority remain undiagnosed and therefore untreated, despite the fact that this serious disorder can have significant consequences like high blood pressure, congestive heart failure, impotency, weight gain, and headaches. Something else scary is that untreated sleep apnea could cause accidents at work or car wrecks from being sleep deprived and sleepy during the day. Fortunately, sleep apnea can be diagnosed and treated. Several treatment options exist. Sometimes, this is in the form of a mask called a cpap that holds the airway open, surgery to remove extra tissues, and even sewing a tennis ball to your pajama back to prevent you from rolling onto your back.

Which came first, "The chicken or the egg?"… I sometimes wonder if obesity causes sleep apnea or if sleep apnea causes obesity. Either way it should always be addressed in any weight loss program.

Some people have a hard time going or staying asleep. You may need to address something called sleep hygiene.

Adrenals, ovaries and testes… Oh my!

So often, I have patients tell me they had their steroid hormone levels checked and they were told they were "fine." My first response is, "If you are 'fine,' then why are you having

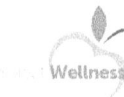
symptoms?" My next question is what reference range were they using? An estrogen level in a little girl is much different than an adult female. An adult menstruating female has different hormone levels than a postmenopausal lady, right? So many times women tell me their doctor said they were in menopause so "of course their hormone levels are low"; like it's normal. But, I assure you, it isn't. If you want to feel like you are in your twenties or thirties, you can't have the hormone levels of a sixty or seventy-year-old female.

What is normal, really? If you have ever seen a range of averages plotted out on a bell curve, you know that you can be on the low end or the high end and still be part of the curve. But if you are having symptoms and on one extreme end of the bell curve or the other, then are you really normal and maybe your body operates at a higher level maximally, but this will not be reflected on an average's curve. We know that levels that are normal in your youth may not be levels that are present after organs like your ovaries fail. So it may be normal not to have much sex steroid hormone around after menopause, according to the numbers game, but does that mean that you will feel like you did when the levels were higher? Probably not.

You are smarter than that. You are proactive and we are all looking for the fountain of youth. Well, it may not be magical or overnight, but we can restore balance and feel better.

When we think about youthful hormones, the steroid or sex hormones are first and foremost. Why? Because when you are at the time in your life when you peak sexually, it is the time you feel the best.

Generally, the steroid hormones come from the reproductive organs. In females, these are the ovaries; and in males, these are the testes. The body has an amazing ability to secure backup plans, and the backup production of these hormones is from the

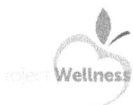

adrenal glands. These little organs sit on top of your kidneys and produce stress hormones and hormones of your fluid and electrolyte balance. It is because of the adrenal production of sex/steroid hormones that you have any sex hormones after menopause.

The steroid hormones are grouped into five main categories by the receptors that they bind to. These are glucocorticoids, mineralocorticoids, androgens (testosterone), estrogens, and progestagens.

From a simplistic point of view, each of these hormones produces certain effects. Some of them you can see, like hair growth or a menstrual cycle. Some you can't see, like internal balance mechanisms.

Oftentimes, I tell women in my practice, I know what they need to adjust based on the symptoms they tell me they are having more than a blood test will ever tell me.

What are designer "bio-identical hormones"?

They are the hormones that are identical to the human body's hormones. When the word "designer" is brought in for discussion, we are talking about the fact that one size does not fit all. The doses are tailored to our individual needs. People need different clothes sizes; our human hormones can vary quite a bit. Even environments affect our hormones through different levels of stress.

The questionnaire I have my patients fill out is quite lengthy, but it helps me to understand them better and how to dose their hormone replacement adequately.

To help you assess the severity of your hormone imbalance, addressing the following list of symptoms or issues may help you

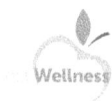

monitor and keep track of your hormone balance. This is a simple checklist that is helpful for patients, I have them check the box if they are having symptoms and then record Mild, Moderate, or Severe after the response.

[] PMS(premenstrual syndrome) issues… cramps, nausea, breast tenderness, headaches, and/or irritability 1-2 weeks before my period

[] Difficulty falling asleep or staying asleep

[] Fatigue or loss of energy especially in the afternoon

[] Frequent bouts of irritability and depression

[] Frequent anxious feelings, anxiety attacks, or heart palpitations

[] Achy or stiff joints, especially in the morning

[] Gaining weight, especially around the middle

[] Losing weight is more difficult than in the past

[] Pain with intercourse

[] Inability to have orgasm, decreased sensitivity, or decreased sex drive

[] Vaginal dryness

[] Crave sweets, carbohydrates or alcohol.

[] Hair or skin that is dry, fragile, or thinning

[] Losing inches of height, diagnosed with osteoporosis, suffered from broken or fractured bones.

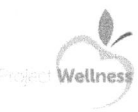

[] Recurrent yeast or urinary tract infections.

[] Irregular menstrual periods.

[] Hot flashes or night sweats.

[] Missing the outer third of your eyebrows

[] Frequent headaches or migraines

[] Fluid retention (rings fit tight or shoe size increased)

[] History of cysts on ovaries

[] Male distribution hair growth (facial hair, male pattern balding)

[] Problems with acne or rosacea

[] Heart racing or irregular heart beats felt

[] Hot or cold intolerance

[] Constipation or diarrhea

[] Frequent bouts of abdominal bloating or gas

[] Skin rashes or new onset allergies

Bioidentical hormones are manufactured in the lab to have the same molecular structure as the hormones made by your own body. By contrast, synthetic hormones are intentionally different. Drug companies can't patent a bioidentical structure, so they invent synthetic hormones that are patentable.

It's so unbelievable to me that bioidentical hormones have been around for years, although most doctors have never heard of them.

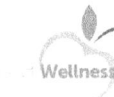
Big pharmaceutical companies who have expensive patented synthetic hormones would like to make sure they never do. The biggest problem is that one size does not fit all when it comes to hormone therapy, and most of the traditional synthetic hormone therapies are only that. One or two, maybe three different doses.

By contrast, the bioidentical or designer hormones are dosed specifically to a patient's blood or saliva hormone levels but mostly by symptoms or concerns. It's important to have your doctor order lab tests (saliva or blood) to establish baselines, rule out serious disease/tumors, and to assess success of absorption into the system from time to time. Not every person needs hormone therapy. When they do though, many medical studies suggest that bioidentical hormones are safer than synthetic versions. It is often possible to rebalance hormones without the use of hormonal supplementation by using nutritional supplements, gentle endocrine support, and dietary and lifestyle changes.

Even with this foundation, a minority of women will need to add prescription-strength hormone supplements to get complete relief, at least through a transition period. We recommend they use bioidentical hormones, preferably in a compounded form personalized to their needs by an experienced practitioner.

There is no substance we introduce into our bodies that is not without potential side effects. Even water can be dangerous when you drink too much. There has been a lot of press around the negative statements from the WHI (women's health initiative) studies on the effectiveness and health risks of HRT, but it is important to remember that these studies were based on synthetic/equine-based hormones that were taken by mouth.

The WHI was launched in 1991 and consisted of a set of clinical trials and an observational study, which together involved 161,808 generally healthy postmenopausal women. The clinical trials were designed to test the effects of postmenopausal hormone therapy,

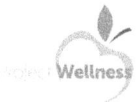

diet modification, and calcium and vitamin D supplements on heart disease, fractures, and breast and colorectal cancer. The hormone trial had two studies: the estrogen-plus-progestin study of women with a uterus, and the estrogen-alone study of women without a uterus. In both hormone therapy studies, women were randomly assigned to either the hormone medication being studied or to placebo.

I personally feel the benefits of bioidentical natural hormone therapy are more than just symptom relief. I rarely run into a woman who is not symptomatic from some sort of hormonal imbalance symptoms; regardless, I feel the benefits of preventing osteoporosis and keeping the mind, skin, and blood vessels youthful is of upmost importance.

With all the controversy around hormones and breast cancer, the question comes up, "What about bioidentical hormones if a person has had breast cancer?"

The pendulum has swung so far that very few doctors will prescribe any type of HRT, synthetic or bioidentical, for women who have had breast cancer or even a family history of breast cancer. I recommend you read Dr. John Lee's book, *What Your Doctor May Not Tell You About Breast Cancer*. He also has several other great books that I consider to be my "bibles" of hormone education study.

Not all estrogens are alike…

Estrogen often gets a "bad rap" because of synthetic versions.

Premenopausal women produce three biologically active estrogens, estrone (E1), estradiol (E2), and estriol (E3). Estradiol is the most abundant estrogen produced and both estrone and estradiol are potent estrogens. Estriol is considered a weak estrogen. Although little scientific data supports the claim, it has been postulated that

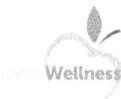

estrone is a "bad" estrogen and may be the cause of estrogen's cancer-causing properties, while estriol is a "good" estrogen and may protect against cancer. Estradiol is probably neutral.

Oral estrogens, not estrogens given by systemic routes (patch, skin cream, vaginal cream, under the tongue), are converted into estrone with potential negative effects for the patient. Oral estrogens, because they are metabolized by the liver, likely exert different effects than systemic estrogens which are not metabolized by the liver.

So, yes, women who have had breast cancer might consider this alternative if they are symptomatic with menopause or pre-menopause. It is thought estrone is a "bad" estrogen and may be the cause of estrogen's cancer-causing properties. Estradiol is probably neutral, but helps significantly with hot flashes.

Over 13 million women were on some form of synthetic HRT before the initial studies were published. When the studies came out millions quit "cold turkey." I can only imagine all those women and their symptoms returning. Many stayed on synthetic HRT but live in fear of the consequences and hormone replacement therapy side effects. Many of those women were unnecessarily placed on antidepressants as pharmaceutical companies and doctors gained alliance to position those drugs as substitute products for lack of hormone balance. Most of these women were not depressed and now have been exposed to a new set of potential side effects.

The majority of studies published to date have concerned synthetic HRT, specifically Premarin and Prempro. Both of these forms are usually take in pill form or orally. Studies have shown levels of CRP (c-reactive protein) are increased with intake of oral estrogen. CRP is a pro-inflammatory blood protein associated with increased risk of heart attack and stroke. Very few have involved or reported anything about bioidentical hormone replacement therapy. Oral

114

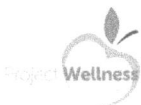

estrogens are converted into estrone with potential negative effects; not estrogens given by transdermal or through the skin routes (patch, skin cream, vaginal cream, under the tongue).

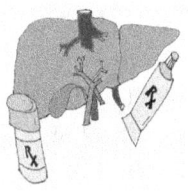

Why creams and gels?

Oral hormones, with a focus on estrogen, are metabolized by the liver. This is known as first pass metabolism. When this happens a normal process occurs that creates "inflammatory proteins." These proteins can cause many different types of inflammation in the body. Of most concern are the blood vessels with a risk of a heart attack or a stroke.

When a route through the skin is chosen, this first pass metabolism by the liver is bypassed and goes straight to the tissues that need it.

This is why we choose creams and gels.

Although I do not recommend oral estrogen, there were problems with the WHI study that no one really talks about. For one thing, the women in the WHI studies were on HRT after menopause while the most common therapeutic use of HRT is for perimenopausal symptoms. Also, the higher risks are small in absolute terms, the increases in relative risk are significant. To take heart attack as one example, the WHI data taken as a whole indicated that out of 10,000 women on Prempro, an extra six would have a heart attack each year compared to women not on Prempro. That may not seem like a substantial risk, but it is a much greater relative risk. The WHI study indicated that the overall increase for women on Prempro for breast cancer was 26%, for

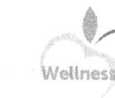
heart attack 29%, for stroke 41%, for blood clots 100%, and for Alzheimer's or dementia over 100%. Many of the top problems in women's health are on that list. And, even if, there is not as great a risk of heart attack as originally supposed, for women closer to menopause, the overall risk-benefit ratio is significant.

Thankfully, there are good alternatives to synthetic HRT. Dr. John Lee, author of *What Your Doctor May Not Tell You About Menopause*, a pioneer of bioidentical hormone therapy stated that there are three rules to hormone replacement therapy. The first rule is to use hormones only if you "need" them (based on lab values or symptoms). The second rule is to use bioidentical hormones and never synthetic, and the third rule is to only use hormone replacement in dosages that create hormone balance. Many women don't even require hormone therapy. Sometimes symptoms can be controlled by a program of core nutritional and endocrine support.

Many women who switch over from oral synthetic estrogen to natural forms of estrogen and progesterone undergo a transition period. It is as if the body's hormone receptors have been primed by the synthetic molecules and have trouble recognizing other forms, even a woman's own. Sometimes, the transition can take four to six weeks. I often start slowly reducing the synthetic dose (not quitting cold turkey from the oral form) as I start with a low dose of bioidentical estrogen and titrate up slowly as the synthetic is getting out of the system. If you stop too abruptly, you may experience extreme hot flashes or other symptoms may flare due to the change in the hormone receptor status.

There are a number of nutritional supplements available that can be extremely helpful in this process. A medical-grade multivitamin combined with calcium, magnesium, and essential fatty acid (fish oil) is critical in diminishing the number and severity of symptoms that occur while one is stopping HRT and afterward. Regular

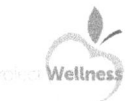

exercise can make a huge difference in terms of the number and intensity of postmenopauseal or perimenopausal symptoms.

The use of Rhubarb plant (I love the estrovera product by Metagenics) and black cohosh as well as soy (80–100 mg of isoflavones a day) may also help abate the symptoms of hot flashes. Be sure to avoid genetically modified soy; choose products labeled "Non-GMO." Soy has also been shown to be helpful in reducing the risk of heart disease; some studies have demonstrated improved bone density, and most recently, studies have shown its ability to decrease the response of insulin in the body, which is particularly important for those who are insulin resistant or diabetic.

Of concern for me is the fact that Wyeth, the manufacturer of Premarin and Prempro, petitioned the FDA in 2005 to restrict the availability of compounded "bio-identical" hormones.

I am grateful several, well-known celebrities have done a lot towards increasing awareness of bio-identical hormones. In 2009, Oprah Winfrey said menopause caught her "off guard" and that taking bioidentical hormones made a big improvement in how she felt. Oprah, when in her mid-fifties, wrote in *O, The Oprah Magazine* that she felt "out of kilter" and had "issues" for two years she suspected were hormonal. Upon a friend's recommendation, Winfrey went to a doctor who specialized in bioidentical hormone therapy. She noted after one day feeling like a veil was lifted. Oprah has done a lot to encourage women to "take charge of their health" and "start the conversation" about menopause and bioidentical hormones.

Suzanne Somers has done a lot to bring information out about bioidenitcal hormones as well. She has written several books and sings the praises of natural hormone therapy. *The Sexy Years,* by Suzanne Somers, delivers helpful information about hormonal imbalances that menopause can bring and she has put bioidentical

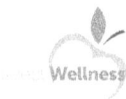
hormones on the map with media appearances on many shows from Home Shopping Network to the Larry King Show.

There are a few things you should know about bioidentical hormones. One of them is that they are usually compounded. This means that they are formulated based on the precise specifications of a doctor who prescribes them. There are many medications that are compounded; bioidentical hormones are just one of the many. Some people say that there is an issue with compounded prescriptions and that they are not FDA approved.

The FDA doesn't approve any compounded products, for any condition, because those products can't be standardized. And, therein lays the beauty in the art of compounding. One size does not fill all when it comes to hormone therapy. I prescribe the lowest and most exact dose formula on symptoms to control those symptoms most effectively. Compounding can also be useful for patients who are allergic to an additive in an FDA-approved product. Because compounded products don't go through the FDA approval process, they don't bear the same warnings as other hormone therapy.

Just because the process is not approved does not mean the actual ingredients are not approved. They absolutely are. It is important that since compounding is a precise science that patients look for accredited compounding pharmacies listed on the web site of the Pharmaceutical Compounding Accreditation Board (PCAB). Since these accredited pharmacies can be hard to find, due to the stringent rules, patients should ask compounding pharmacies what types of quality assurance procedures are in place. Also, you will need to ask for information on side effects and warnings because these may not be included when prescriptions are compounded.

It is not completely necessary you use compounded hormones. There are FDA-approved "bioidentical" drugs available. The biggest reason for using compounding is the customization of doses. Another reason to use compounding would be if someone

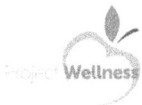

has allergies to ingredients, or intolerances to doses, in commercially available products.

There is no reason to think bioidentical compounded products would have a different safety profile than the FDA-approved ones. You must be careful as some compounding pharmacies have gotten warning letters from the FDA for false and misleading claims about safety and other benefits.

Compounding pharmacies can formulate products into many forms including tablets, capsules, creams, gels, lozenges, suppositories, and more. Compounding pharmacies create products from one or more active ingredients. The United States Pharmacopeia (USP) is the recognized national formulary and offers guidance for compounding. Ingredients, according to the USP, must meet quality standards, such as pharmaceutical grade, reagent grade, or even food grade. The active ingredients and inactive ingredients are specified by a licensed health care physician with a prescription.

The healthcare practitioner specifies ingredients and doses intended to meet the individual needs of their patients. For example, these pharmacies can combine multiple bioidentical hormones of various strengths into one compounded medication. The prescriber will also specify the type of formulation to use. Flavoring can be added to formulations to make them more palatable if desired.

The greatest success comes from an individualized approach. When warranted, we prescribe a precise dosage of bioidentical estrogen, testosterone, or DHEA that is made up at a compounding pharmacy to alleviate individual symptoms and target specific issues to the individual. Each patient is then monitored carefully through regular follow-up. Treatment and adjustments should be based on symptoms and quality of life issues more than blood hormone levels. Lab tests (saliva or blood) are best to use to

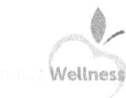

establish baselines, rule out serious disease/tumors, and to assess
success of absorption into the system.

I get asked many times, "How long will I need to be on hormone
therapy?"

The answer to this depends on how long you have symptoms or the
body has issues consistent with hormone deficiencies. For some,
this is a few months—for others, many years.

I also get asked about having periods after menopause. It is not
necessary for a postmenopausal woman to have periods if she is
using bioidentical hormones properly. When postmenopausal
women use small doses of bioidentical hormones, they rarely, if
ever, have periods. Nor do they have the risky endometrial
buildup in the uterus, which is what makes it important to have
periods. Estrogen stimulates the buildup of uterine tissue, but
there's no need to take that much estrogen to feel healthy and
balanced. Since fat cells create estrogen, women who are heavy
may not even need to use supplemental estrogen.

Dr. Lee's recommendation was always to use the lowest dose
possible of any hormone supplementation. Usually this was 15 to
30 mg of progesterone daily, and the lowest dose of estrogen that
would either clear up estrogen deficiency symptoms or show
normal levels on a saliva hormone level test. This improves health
and well being but doesn't put a postmenopausal woman back into
the same hormonal milieu she had when she was menstruating
every month.

When you take progesterone in a pill form, most of it goes directly
to the liver, where up to 80 percent of it may be dumped, but not
before creating a variety of byproducts (metabolites). Thus, it's
necessary to take 100 mg of progesterone in pill form to get 20 mg
into your cells. If your liver happens to be working less efficiently
on a given day and excretes less of the progesterone, it's easy to

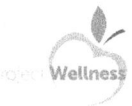

experience overdose side effects, such as sleepiness and bloating. These side effects often have women running for more estrogen to wake themselves up again. What they really need to do is use progesterone cream, which is a much more efficient delivery method. If you put 20 mg on your skin, virtually all of that will be in your bloodstream within a matter of minutes.

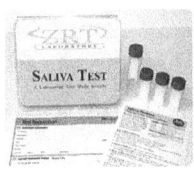 Saliva Testing? What's that all about?

Saliva testing has become the most specific way to assess the hormone levels in your tissues. Blood tests show only fluctuating levels from minute to minute. A full assessment of multiple hormones can be tested. It is easy to do. Although some insurance does not pay for it, these tests can be more affordable than blood tests in some cases.

Saliva testing is a convenient, inexpensive, and above all, accurate means of testing steroid hormones. Scientific studies have shown a strong correlation between steroid hormone levels in saliva, and the amount of hormone in the blood that is active or "bioavailable." Saliva is an ideal diagnostic medium to measure the bioavailable levels of steroid hormones active in the tissue. It is this fraction of total hormone that is free to enter the target tissues in the brain, uterus, skin, and breasts.

Saliva testing can be done anywhere, anytime. Testing that relies on blood drawn in the doctor's office makes it harder to obtain samples at specific times (such as in the early morning) or multiple times during the day. In addition, hormones in saliva are exceptionally stable and can be stored at room temperature for up to a week without affecting the accuracy of the result. This offers maximum flexibility in sample collection and shipment. Several of the steroid hormones can be tested in the saliva including,

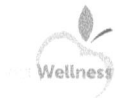
estradiol, estrone, estriol, progesterone, testosterone, DHEA-S, and cortisol.

When a woman experiences prolonged stress, pregnenolone (that comes from the precursor cholesterol), a hormone essential for both coping with stress and producing female hormones, is diverted from the normal hormone pathway. As a result, the production of female hormones is compromised. This condition can cause a multitude of symptoms including irritability, mood swings, headaches, sleeplessness, and weight gain.

Each person is different, and the whole person and hormonal chemical make-up and balance are unique.  The doctor must take into account all the different complexities of an individual's hormone make-up and balance and work with what the person has in their environment to maximize the hormonal balance.

The hormonal health of any woman depends upon the delicate dance of progesterone and estrogen. Estrogen is meant to be the predominant hormone in the first half of the menstrual cycle, and progesterone the predominant one in the second half. However, for most women in the industrialized world, this is not the case.

There are many causes of hormone imbalance, but at the base of the problem is something called Estrogen Dominance, which means there is too much estrogen and not enough progesterone present in the body. There are many symptoms that result from having low progesterone levels.

What follows is a look at some of the common ways in which medicine and industry have tampered with the natural balance of our hormones. Women have used these products blindly at the cost of our hormonal balance, overall health, and longevity. Some of these may be obvious to you, while some may come as a surprise. Either way the hormonal imbalances that result should not be taken

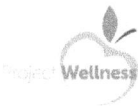

lightly. They contribute to the rise in cancers, especially breast and ovarian cancers, heart disease, depression, PMS, and more.

The common causes of hormonal imbalance and estrogen dominance:

- Artificial hormone replacement therapy (The Pill and Prempro)
- Environmental poisons
- Non organic and estrogen pumped animal products
- Stress
- Cosmetics (chemicals in them that mimic estrogen in the body)

Progestins and progestogens (artificial progesterone) are highly toxic to the body, resulting in some of these known side effects:

- miscarriages
- migraines
- heart disease
- high blood pressure
- cancer
- depression

and, of course … low progesterone, the true biologic levels.

These are some of the common ways that medicine has tampered with the natural balance of hormones, here are some the ways that industry has tampered with the same delicate hormonal balance.

Chemicals such as pesticides mimic the hormone estrogen. Fifty-one chemicals have now been identified as hormone disruptors. Approximately 2 billion tons of pesticides are used annually. In undeveloped countries, the use of pesticides is still largely unchecked and … guess what?  That is where we get a lot of our food supplies. It's plain to see why this is wreaking havoc on our bodies. It is this fact that has led many people to switch to an organic diet.

Other chemicals that cause the same challenges are DDT, dioxin, and PCBs (polychlorinated biphenyls). Dioxin is the byproduct of the manufacture of chemicals using chlorine and includes:

- disinfectants
- dry cleaning fluids
- pesticides
- drugs
- plastics, like polystyrene and ClingWrap

PCBs are used in:

- lubricants
- plastics
- paints
- varnishes
- inks

Commonly called petrochemicals, they contain high levels of xeno-estrogens. Xeno-estrogens basically mean they mimic estrogen in your body. They fill up all the estrogen receptor sites in your body; even the good estrogen can't get through to perform its role properly. This results in hormone imbalance.  This is why many people have moved over to household cleaning products that don't contain these chemicals and are environmentally friendly. Non-organic animals that are slaughtered for our food chain are fed estrogenic steroids to fatten them up. These estrogens go straight into our bloodstream causing a further rise in estrogen levels. Another study linked the increase of our current disease rates to eating a diet high in the fat and meat from these estrogen-fed animals. Again, it is this fact that has led many people to switch to an organic diet.  Cosmetics may come as a surprise to you, but

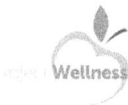

many cosmetics are made with petrochemicals. Yes, like the kind you put in your car. It's not surprising then to realize that these "moisturizers" are actually drying out your skin—actually causing more wrinkles!

Even more importantly, they are putting your hormones further out of balance. Just to list a few: aqueous cream, petroleum jelly, mineral oil, liquid paraffin, talc powders, parabens, and other estrogenic antioxidants.

Again, this is why many people have moved over to moisturizers that don't contain these chemicals and are environmentally friendly.

As if all of the above were not enough, stress also plays a big part in reducing our levels of progesterone, which actually results in *too much* estrogen.

Here's how: Progesterone is the "mother of all hormones." It is the precursor and essential raw material out of which the body created ALL THE OTHER HORMONES. As the precursor to all the other hormones in the body, the adrenal glands and adrenal hormones are no exception. If you encounter a mildly stressful situation, your body draws on its progesterone to produce the hormones (adrenal corticosteroids) to counteract it. These are the hormones that protect against stress. But if your body is in a constant state of stress, it can't provide enough progesterone to be converted into anti-stress hormones, and the result is adrenal exhaustion and no left over progesterone for other normal body functions. You can change your life! You can restore balance. You can combat aging and ill health effects starting today. You must find someone knowledgeable about hormones who will listen to you and your situation and find the right solution that fits only you.

Bioidentical hormones are already in our bodies. I have patients who need oxygen supplementation often tell me that they are afraid

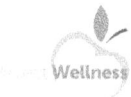

they will get "addicted" to oxygen if they start using a machine. This is so silly because we are all addicted to oxygen. We need it every second of every day. The same holds true with our hormones. We need them every second of every day and using natural hormones to supplement deficiencies cannot possibly cause you to become addicted to hormones. I am always careful to use the term supplementation, not replacement. You do not simply stop making sex steroid hormones after your ovaries fail and shrivel up. You still make hormones from your adrenal glands, the little guys on top of the kidneys, although, in much smaller amounts than if you have healthy active ovaries. Supplementing your body to bring you back in balance only makes sense in many circumstances.

The process of aging is accompanied by reduced levels of hormones that maintain our youth. With this decline, heart disease, stroke, osteoporosis, chronic inflammatory, and neurodegenerative disorders develop in both men and women.

Men have problems with decreasing testosterone as well. Mainstream medicine's ignorance regarding the need to maintain testosterone in the higher ranges is a significant cause of premature disability and death in aging men. Most people are in a state of denial about declining hormone levels. A man between 30 and 40 years is often shocked when his blood test results uncover strikingly low testosterone levels. I see it in my practice all the time, especially if they are overweight.

HDL is the "good cholesterol" and protects against atherosclerosis and heart disease. Testosterone plays a critical role in helping HDL to remove the built-up bad cholesterol away from the arterial wall.

Testosterone is required for optimal transport of excess cholesterol from our tissues and blood vessels to our liver for processing and

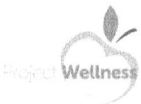

disposal. In the testosterone-deficient state, reverse cholesterol transport is compromised, and excess cholesterol cannot be removed from the arterial wall.

One of the biggest barriers for testosterone supplementation is the fear of prostate cancer. However, this need not be a fear because hundreds of clinical trials have shown that low testosterone is more of a risk factor for prostate cancer than high testosterone levels, and men with low testosterone levels have an increased percentage of prostate cancer-positive biopsies. It has been shown that as free testosterone levels decline in aging men, their PSA levels sharply increase. Even though it is clear that testosterone does not cause prostate cancer, I still advise avoidance of testosterone until the disease is cured in a male with active untreated diagnosed prostate cancer.

Another problem with hormonal imbalance is that excess abdominal fat is a major culprit in many men with high estradiol levels. Excess body fat, particularly in the abdominal region, is a major factor in imbalanced estrogen metabolism. Abdominal obesity increases aromatase activity, which increases estradiol, which in excess causes more abdominal fat. A negative feedback loop is established and health suffers as a result. Reducing abdominal fat will mitigate excessive estradiol levels. Zinc is very helpful in the process of reversing this loop. Wheat germ is an excellent, high-potency vegetarian source of zinc.

Zinc also functions as an aromatase inhibitor in many men. Although red meats are a primary source of zinc, non-meat sources such as wheat germ or roasted pumpkin and squash seeds compare quite favorably with the levels found in animal protein sources. For estradiol balance, zinc can be supplemented at 80mg per day. DIM (di-indolmethane) is derived from the phytochemical IC3 (Indole-3-Carbinol). DIM works by converting estradiol into a less potent, and less harmful, form of estrogen called estriol. Although both DIM and IC3 can be found in nutrient supplement forms, IC3 is also found naturally in cruciferous vegetables such as cabbage, broccoli, and kale. In supplement form, DIM is more easily absorbed into the body.

In males, the main biologically active estrogen is estradiol. The primary source of estradiol in men is from the conversion (aromatization) of testosterone. As men age, the production of androgens from the adrenals and gonads is decreased. The aromatization of testosterone to estradiol is often maintained, but due to a variety of factors, more testosterone is aromatized in fatty tissues, causing a further imbalance of the ratio of testosterone to estrogen, i.e. too much estradiol and not enough testosterone. The result is a deficiency of beneficial testosterone and an excess amount of estradiol.

As men age, the amount of testosterone produced in the testes diminishes greatly, yet estradiol levels remain persistently high. The reason for this is increasing aromatase activity along with age-associated fat mass, especially in the belly.

Estradiol levels correlate significantly to body fat mass and more specifically to subcutaneous abdominal fat. The epidemic of abdominal obesity observed in aging men is associated with a constellation of degenerative disorders, including heart disease, diabetes, and cancer.

Subcutaneous abdominal fat acts as a secretory gland, often producing and emitting excessive levels of estradiol into an aging man's blood. One's waist circumference is a highly accurate prognostic measurement of future disease risk. Excess estradiol secretion is at least one of the deadly mechanisms associated with the difficult-to-resolve problem of having too much abdominal fat. Symptoms of excess estrogen in aging men include the development of breasts, having too much abdominal weight, feeling tired, suffering loss of muscle mass, and having emotional disturbances. Many of these symptoms correspond to testosterone deficiency as well.

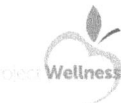 

Both men and women need estrogen to maintain bone density, cognitive function, and even to maintain the inner lining of the arterial wall (the endothelium). Both men and women with declining hormone levels are at increased risk of osteoporosis, a condition that means your bones are weak, and you're more likely to break a bone. Since there are no symptoms, you might not know your bones are getting weaker until you break a bone. A broken bone can cause disability, pain, or loss of independence.

With the decline of the female hormone estrogen at menopause, usually around age 50, bone breakdown markedly increases. For several years, women lose bone two to four times faster than they did before menopause. The rate usually slows down again, but some women may continue to lose bone rapidly. By age 65, some women have lost half their skeletal mass.

The FDA has approved several kinds of devices that use various methods to estimate bone density. A newer technique for evaluating bone strength is ultrasound, and the FDA has approved several instruments for this purpose. The devices for ultrasound measurement are cheaper and easier to use. This makes them available in more locations and allows evaluation for osteoporosis in many more subjects. Another new test provides an indicator of bone breakdown. In 1995, the FDA approved a simple, noninvasive biochemical test that detects in a urine sample a specific component of bone breakdown, called NTx.

Calcium and vitamin D supplements are an integral part of all treatments for osteoporosis. Healthy diet and exercise are important not only for treatment, but also for prevention. A lifelong habit of weight-bearing exercise, such as walking or biking, also helps build and maintain strong bone. The greatest benefit for older people is that physical fitness reduces the risk of fracture. Better balance, muscle strength, and agility make falls less likely. People who don't consume dairy foods can meet their calcium needs with foods that are fortified with calcium, such as orange juice, or with calcium supplements. Other good sources of calcium are dark-green leafy vegetables like kale and turnip greens, tofu (if made with calcium), canned fish (eaten with bones), and fortified cereal products. Women over the age of 50 should have at least 1200 mg/day and women from 19-50 should have about 1,000 mg.

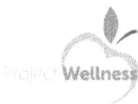
Thyroid Hormone:

The thyroid gland sits in your mid neck, is shaped like a butterfly, and consists of two lobes that lie on each side of the trachea (windpipe) located just below the Adam's apple. It's one of the largest endocrine glands in the body and is also one of the most amazing and sensitive. This unique mass of specialized tissue produces the thyroid hormones thyroxine (T4) and triiodothyronine (T3), the primary regulators of human metabolism. The numbers 4 & 3 after the "T" designate the number of iodine atoms they each contain. Both hormones are derived from the amino acid tyrosine. Thyroid hormones accelerate cellular reactions and increase oxidative metabolism, by stimulating enzymes that control active transport pumps, demand for cellular oxygen increases, and as ATP production goes up and heat is produced. This creates a thermoregulatory effect, which increases body temperature.

Basal metabolic rate (BMR) is directly influenced by thyroid hormone biochemistry. Thyroid hormones can target, influence, and alter the metabolism of virtually every cell in the body. They affect mood, bodyweight, stamina, and even fertility. Thyroid hormones stimulate protein synthesis and increase the rate at which triglycerides are broken down (lipolysis) affecting the appearance of the body's muscle physique and help preserve muscle and reduce body fat. When used incorrectly and/or excessively, they are highly catabolic to muscle or have the opposite effect. This is why it is not recommended to use thyroid supplementation just for aesthetics, it is too difficult to overuse and have the reverse of what you want and why it is important to monitor levels in the blood to achieve desired results.

Synthetic forms of pure thyroxine (Synthroid, Levothroid, Levoxyl) rate high on the list of drugs most frequently prescribed by physicians. They can stimulate appetite, speed metabolic rate and help people lose weight. But if abused or used incorrectly, they can also cause serious heart problems, muscle weakness, and muscle wasting. Alternatives to T4 alone include synthetic T3 (Cytomel) and desiccated animal gland extracts that contain both T4 & T3 (Armour, Naturthroid, Westroid). All forms may be useful depending on the individual and thyroid condition. The solution is to determine the best dose, form, and combination.

The thyroid secretes about 10 times as much T4 as T3; however, T3 is roughly 2-3 times more potent. Thyroxine is converted into the more active triiodothyronine with the selenium dependent enzyme 5'-deiodinase. Thus, some thyroid disorders are simply a consequence of consuming a diet that lacks sufficient selenium. T3 and T4 are lipid-soluble and combine with special transport proteins upon release into the serum, called thyroxine-binding globulins (TBG). Less than 1% of thyroid hormones travel unattached in their free state.

During growth, thyroid hormones provide an anabolic influence on protein metabolism. This is due to their influence on insulin secretion. T4 and insulin also connect in the liver, where they mutually affect IGF activity. IGF (Insulin Growth Factors) are powerful muscle building control agents. In the absence of adequate levels of thyroid hormones, human growth hormone (hGH) also loses its growth-promoting action and is not secreted normally.

Thyroid problems are incredibly common in North America, especially among women. As a rule, when all else fails and you can't figure out what's wrong, suspect low thyroid and get it tested ASAP. Many experts believe this epidemic is caused by excess chemicals in our food, air, and water. All of these stress the immune system leading to a high incidence of autoimmune illness. Common symptoms of low thyroid include unusual fatigue, susceptibility to feeling cold, trouble with weight management, prominent bags under eyes, muscle and joint aches and pains, problems with digestion, mental sluggishness, dry skin, depression,

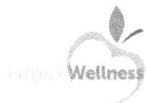
migraines, and waking up feeling tired. Instead of feeling refreshed after a morning workout, you might feel like going back to bed (even though it's only 10 a.m.). Or, after work instead of heading to the gym, you head straight home because you feel completely drained. Athletes with low thyroid do not perform well when the ambient temperature drops below 50° F. The synovial fluid in the joints also tends to "thicken," thus reducing joint motility and increasing risk of injury.

Women typically under consume protein, especially low-fat, non-denatured animal protein, which provides a strong source of the essential amino acid phenylalanine. Tyrosine is known as the "anti-stress" amino and is greatly depleted after hard workouts and exhausting sport competition. Thyroid hormones depend on ample pools of tyrosine, which is dependent on phenylalanine intake. Fortunately, tyrosine can be taken directly in supplement form.

Women are prone to anemia or iron deficiency through menstrual cycles, which can exacerbate thyroid problems because iron influences thyroid function. Anemia induced through iron deficiency has been shown to significantly reduce circulating levels of T4-5'deiodinase, resulting in suppression of the conversion of T4 to T3 thereby resulting in low plasma T4 levels. After 12 weeks of iron supplementation and iron deficiency correction, both T4 levels and the ability of the body to thermoregulate body temperature following exposure to cold improves.

The thyroid gland is the main metabolic regulator of our bodies. To convert thyroxine (T4) the inactive form to triiodthyronine (T3), the active form requires the removal of an iodine molecule from T4, and adequate stores of iodine are needed to then make more T4. This process also requires the mineral selenium, vitamin A, vitamin E, zinc, and iron, and without them can imitate iodine deficiency.

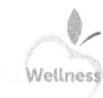

Some symptoms of iodine deficiency are cognitive impairment, fibrocystic breast disease, goiter, hyperthyroidism, hypothyroidism, and miscarriages.

So many times have I heard, "My doctor tested my thyroid and it was fine." The problem is many people recognize that the thyroid regulates metabolism, but are not educated or empowered enough to go one step further. To this day, I do not understand why so many doctors think that TSH (thyroid stimulating hormone) blood tests are the only way to diagnose thyroid problems. When I was an X-ray tech, we were taught that "one view was no view." This meant that when we did an X-ray of a chest, only using a front to back view was not enough information. You had to do a side view as well. We called this a 2-view chest. You can't see through the tissues the other way, and the same was with extremities like arms and legs. You might miss a fracture if you didn't get the other views or angles. Well, lab testing is the same way. One test is NO test! You have to have the rest of the information to make a diagnosis to see the whole picture. You have to understand what the tests mean, too. You must also recognize that "normal" values are a bell curve or an average of patients tested who are "normal." Does that mean if you are one point outside the range that suddenly you are "abnormal?" This is crazy to think such an arbitrary cutoff can make you normal or abnormal or rule out disease.

Many endocrinologists (specialists who deal with hormonal issues) are known for being "numbers" people. They manage by the numbers, and not by the symptoms. This method can often create the "you're in the normal range, so you're fine" response from doctors when many of us complain we still don't feel well. Keep in mind, if you have easily diagnosed hypothyroidism, it may take some serious looking to find an endocrinologist who believes in finding an optimal TSH for you.

Diagnosing thyroid disease is a process that can incorporate numerous factors, including clinical evaluation, blood tests,

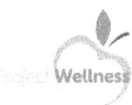

imaging tests, biopsies, and other tests.  Many thyroid diseases exist beyond just a "hypofunctioning" gland.  These include: hypothyroidism, Hashimoto's Disease, hyperthyroidism: Graves' Disease, goiter (enlarged gland), and nodules (lumpy gland).

Here is a list of different blood tests used to diagnose thyroid issues.

- Thyroid Stimulating Hormone (TSH) Test
- Total T4 (Thyroxine)
- Free T4 (Thyroxine)
- Total T3 (Triiodothyronine)
- Free T3 (Triiodothyronine)
- Thyroglobulin (Thyroid Binding Globulin/TBG)
- T3 Resin Uptake (T3RU)
- Reverse T3
- Thyroid Peroxidase Antibodies (TPOAb) (Antithyroid Peroxidase Antibodies)
- Antithyroid Microsomal Antibodies (Antimicrosomal Antibodies)
- Thyroglobulin Antibodies (Antithyroglobulin Antibodies)
- Thyroid Receptor Antibodies (TRAb)
- Thyroid-Stimulating Immunoglobulins (TSI)

TSH blood Test - The most common thyroid test is the blood test that measures the amount of thyroid-stimulating hormone (TSH) in your bloodstream.  Here's where it gets tricky!  If the TSH is elevated or high, we think hypothyroidism or low function.  If the TSH is low, then this is usually evidence of hyperthyroidism.  This may seem a little backwards, but TSH is a hormone from that brain that has a "feedback effect" on the thyroid gland.  So, when the TSH is elevated, you may have a low thyroid function.  When it is low, you may have an overly functioning thyroid.

Free T4 / Free Thyroxine - Free T4 measures the free, unbound
thyroxine levels in your bloodstream. Free T4 is typically elevated
in hyperthyroidism and lowered in hypothyroidism. Free or
unbound T4 levels represent the level of hormone available for
uptake and use by cells. Bound levels represent a circulating
hormone that may not all be immediately available, because it is
affected by other drugs, illness, and physical changes, such as
pregnancy. Because the free levels of T4 represent immediately
available hormone, free T4 is thought to better reflect the patient's
available hormonal status than total T4.

Total T4/Total Thyroxine - This test measures the total amount of
circulating thyroxine in your blood. Thyroxine, a hormone
produced by the thyroid, is also known as T4. A high value can
indicate hyperthyroidism; a low value can indicate
hypothyroidism. Total T4 levels can be elevated due to pregnancy
and other high estrogen states, including use of estrogen
replacement or birth control pills.

Total T3/Total Triiodothyronine - Triiodothyronine is the active
thyroid hormone and is also known as T3. Total T3 is typically
elevated in hyperthyroidism and lowered in hypothyroidism.

Free T3 / Free Triiodothyronine - Free T3 measures the free,
unbound levels of triiodothyronine in your bloodstream. Free T3 is
considered more accurate than Total T3. Free T3 is typically
elevated in hyperthyroidism and lowered in hypothyroidism.

T3 Resin Uptake (T3RU) – Just one more piece of the puzzle. Not
used a lot but when done with a T3 and T4, the T3 resin uptake
(T3RU) test is sometimes referred to as the T7 test. This test
measures the amount of unsaturated binding sites on the transport
(binding) hormones. The T3RU test measures the level of proteins
that carry thyroid hormone in the blood. Elevated T3RU is more
commonly seen with hyperthyroidism. Keep in mind, certain

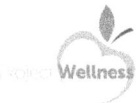
medications like steroids, heparin, phenytoin, aspirin, and Coumadin can increase T3RU values and male androgen replacement, illness and kidney disease can increase thyroxin binding globulin (TBG) levels. There are drugs that can decrease T3RU values like antithyroid medications, birth control pills, clofibrate, estrogen, and thiazides. Pregnancy can also decrease T3RU levels.

Thyroglobulin/Tg - Thyroglobulin (Tg) levels are low or undetectable with normal thyroid function but can by elevated in thyroiditis, Graves' disease, or thyroid cancer. Monitoring of Tg levels is frequently used as a tumor marker to evaluate the effectiveness of treatment for thyroid cancer and to monitor for thyroid cancer recurrence.

Reverse T3 - When the body is under stress, instead of converting T4 into T3 - the active form of thyroid hormone - the body conserves energy by making what is known as Reverse T3 (RT3), an inactive form of the T3 hormone. The value of RT3 tests in diagnosis is controversial, as some practitioners believe that the body continues to manufacture RT3 instead of active T3, causing various symptoms that are identified as Wilson's syndrome or symptomatic low function thyroid issues.

Thyroid Peroxidase (TPO) Antibodies (TPOAb) / Antithyroid Peroxidase Antibodies - Thyroid Peroxidase (TPO) antibodies, are also known as Antithyroid Peroxidase Antibodies. (In the past, these antibodies were referred to as Antithyroid Microsomal Antibodies or Antimicrosomal Antibodies). These antibodies work against thyroid peroxidase, an enzyme that plays a part in the T4-to-T3 conversion and synthesis process. TPO antibodies can be evidence of tissue destruction, such as Hashimoto's disease, less commonly, in other forms of thyroiditis such as post-partum thyroiditis. It's estimated that TPO antibodies are detectable in approximately 95 percent of patients with Hashimoto's thyroiditis

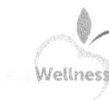
and 50 to 85 percent of Graves' disease patients. The concentrations of antibodies found in patients with Graves' disease are usually lower than in patients with Hashimoto's disease.

Thyroglobulin Antibodies / Antithyroglobulin Antibodies - Testing for thyroglobulin antibodies (also called antithyroglobulin antibodies) is common. If you have already been diagnosed with Graves' disease, having high levels of thyroglobulin antibodies means that you are more likely to eventually become hypothyroid. Thyroglobulin antibodies are positive in about 60 percent of Hashimoto's patients and 30 percent of Graves' patients.

Thyroid-Stimulating Immunoglobulins (TSI) / TSH Stimulating Antibodies (TSAb) - TSH receptor antibodies (TRAb) are seen in most patients with a history of, or who currently have, Graves' disease. Testing is usually done for a specific type of stimulating TRAb that goes by several different names, including:  Thyroid-Stimulating Immunoglobulins (TSI) and TSH stimulating antibodies (TSAb).  Thyroid-stimulating immunoglobulins (TSI) can be detected in the majority - some estimates say as many as 75 to 90 percent - of Graves' disease patients. The higher the levels, the more active the Graves' disease is thought to be. (The absence of these antibodies does not, however, rule out Graves' disease.) Less commonly, some people with Hashimoto's disease also have these antibodies, and this can cause periodic short-term episodes of hyperthyroidism. When monitoring TSI, elevated levels may help predict relapse of Graves' disease, and lowered TSI levels may indicate that Graves' disease treatment is working.

TRH test- If hypothyroidism symptoms are present but TSH tests are normal, the physician measures the patient's TSH level (a simple blood test), gives an injection of TRH, then draws blood 25 minutes later and remeasures the TSH. If the first TSH level is normal and the second TSH level is high (greater than 10) the patient's thyroid is underactive. A TSH reading of 15 is suspicious,

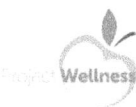

while 20 strongly points to hypothyroidism. If you have three or more typical symptoms of underactive thyroid but have tested 'normal' in standard tests, 35-40% actually have underactive thyroids based on the TRH test

To completely evaluate your thyroid function, your doctor should do the following:

Feel your thyroid gland for lumps, nodules, enlargement, or "thrills," a rushing of blood through it.

Listen to your thyroid using a stethoscope for bruits or sounds of increased blood flow in the thyroid.

Test your reflexes at the knee and ankle with a hammer to see if your reflexes are over or underactive. Hyper-responsive reflexes can be a sign of hyperthyroidism, and slow reflexes may point to hypothyroidism.

Check your heart rate, rhythm, and blood pressure. A slow heart rate (bradycardia) may point to hypothyroidism. A high heart rate (tachycardia), high blood pressure, or rhythm irregularites may point to hyperthyroidism.

Measure your weight. Rapid weight gain, without a change to diet or exercise, can be a sign of hypothyroidism. Rapid weight loss may point to hyperthyroidism.

Measure body temperature. Low body temperature might be a possible sign of an underactive thyroid.

Examine your face, looking for loss of hair in the outer edge of the eyebrows—a symptom of hypothyroidism—as well as puffiness or swelling in the eyelids or face, another common hypothyroidism symptom. The eyes are often affected in thyroid patients. Common clinical symptoms include: bulging or protrusion of the eyes, a stare in the eyes, retraction of upper eyelids, a wide-eyed look, infrequent blinking, and "lid lag"— when the upper eyelid doesn't smoothly follow downward movements of the eyes when you look down.  Dull facial expression, hoarseness, or swelling in the face, hands, or feet can be a sign of thyroid disorder.

Observe the general quantity and quality of your hair as hair loss is seen in both overactive and underactive thyroid. Coarse, brittle, or straw-like hair can point to hypothyroidism. Thinning, finer hair may point to hyperthyroidism.

Examine your skin as thyroid disease, especially hyperthyroidism, can show up in a variety of skin-related symptoms that include yellowish, jaundiced cast to the skin, unusually smooth, young-looking skin, hives, lesions or patches of rough skin on the shins (known as pretibial myxedema or Graves' dermopathy), or blister-like bumps of the forehead and face (known as milaria bumps).

Examine your nails and hands looking for hyperthyroidism related clinical signs in your nails and hands, including: Onycholysis or separation of the nail from the underlying nail bed, also called Plummer's nails, swollen fingertips, or acropachy.

Review other clinical signs of hyperthyroidism, including: tremors, shaky hands, hyperkinetic movements like table drumming, tapping feet, and jerky movements.  Tests that may not be considered thyroid evaluations like bone density (DEXA scan or x-ray) as low bone density may be helpful to evaluate thyroid issues.

Some less mainstream tests that may be used are:

1. Iodine Patch Tests – paint a 1-inch square on your inner arm of iodine and watch to see how long it

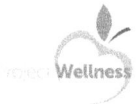

takes to absorb.  Less than 1 hour and you may have an iodine deficiency.

2.  Saliva Testing – for hormones and blood spot

3.  Urinary Testing – for iodine

4.  Basal Body Temperature Testing - Before going to bed at night, place a basal thermometer on your bedside table. As soon as you wake up, place the thermometer in the center of your armpit and then lay still for about 10 minutes. Record your body temperature and repeat this procedure for 3 consecutive days. Women should do this test during the first few days after menstruation begins.  Add the three temperatures together and divide by 3. This figure represents your average basal metabolic temperature, which is reflective of thyroid hormone output. A normal temperature is approximately 37° C (98° F).  Although "normal" does vary from person to person, a reading 1° or more below this range could indicate a problem with your thyroid.

Some patients need to be highly involved in their thyroid diagnosis and care.  Self-tests and the ability to order your own tests can be a critical tool for an empowered patient.

Some things you can do at home to aid in detecting thyroid problems are:

Self neck, thyroid checks.  To do this, hold a mirror up so you can see your thyroid area: the neck, just below the Adam's apple and above the collarbone. Tip your head back and, keeping an eye on this thyroid area, take a drink of water and swallow. As you swallow, look at your neck. Watch carefully for any bulges, enlargement, protrusions, or unusual appearances in this area. Repeat this process several times. If you see any bulges,

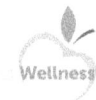

protrusions, lumps, or anything that appears unusual, see your doctor right away.

Get lab testing and don't settle for just a TSH!

Being informed and knowledgeable about thyroid disease signs, symptoms, and risks can be an important part of getting properly diagnosed. Diagnosis of various thyroid disease and conditions involves clinical examination, blood tests, and in some cases, imaging tests and/or biopsy.

So, if you have low functioning thyroid issues, what are your treatment options? Synthroid, Levoxyl, Levothyroid, Euthyrox, Eltroxin are all brand names for the thyroid drug levothyroxine sodium, which is a synthetic version of the thyroid hormone T4. Remember that T4 is the inactive form of thyroid hormone and must be converted to T3. These are the drugs prescribed for thyroid hormone replacement for most patients. If you have hypothyroidism and are taking one of these conventional thyroid replacement drugs, your blood tests show a "normal" TSH, and, yet, you still don't feel well, there may be a need for the addition of T3 or active form of thyroid hormone.

If you have the inability to adequately convert T4 to the T3 needed by the body, you may still have a normal TSH, but present many hypothyroid symptoms. Serum hormone studies typically show marginally low T3 and T4 levels, usually within the "normal" range, and TSH is rarely elevated out of the "normal range." At the same time, cholesterol is often elevated, and basal temperature is likely to be 97 degrees F or less. Patients with hypometabolism problems often respond well to T3 or T4/T3 treatments.

Some scientists believe this may be the underlying cause of fibromylagia symptoms. Researchers have found higher incidence of thyroid disease among fibromylagia patients. And the researchers are also finding these patients need the additional

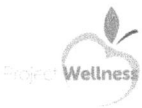
thyroid hormone T3 to resolve symptoms.

T3 is available on its own in compound extended release forms or can be included with T4 in the naturally derived thyroid drug Armour Thyroid.

It is not recommended you use thyroid replacement for weight loss alone. You may make some issues worse or create new issues. If you have symptoms of low thyroid function and are overweight, than to not use some form of thyroid support will leave you spinning your wheels.

You owe it to yourself to understand your thyroid. Here are a few questions you may want to ask yourself.

[]Do you find that no matter how much you sleep, you're always waking up exhausted?

[]Do you feel like you have cobwebs in your head or constant brain fog?

[]Do you feel like even though you watch your diet, cut out junk food and exercise, the scale won't budge or you even gain weight?

[]Do you lose hair or does it feel thinner? Do you see it when you clean out the shower drain?

[]Do you battle depression or anxiety?

[]After childbirth, did you fail to lose "baby weight?"

[]Do you have ice-cold hands or feet?

[]Do you have dry skin?

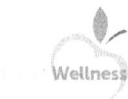

[]Do you have insomnia or a poor sleep quality?

[]Do you have tingling in hands and feet?

[]Do you have muscle pain?

[]Do you have edema (swelling in ankles, legs, or hands)?

[]Do you have elevated cholesterol?

All the symptoms above can be caused by an underactive thyroid or hypothyroidism. It can start as early as our middle twenties, getting progressively worse as we age.

Many people think thyroid when they think tired. So, they go to their doctor and try to talk about it. Your doctor humors you by giving you a thyroid blood test. Of course, when it comes back, you'll be told your thyroid is normal. You'll then be told it's "all in your head" and be given a prescription for anti-depressants. When a lab test is done, any result within a wide range is deemed normal. Your thyroid could be functioning at 30% of peak efficiency, even though it is within that "normal" range.

Taking an anti-depressant won't do a thing for your symptoms or your condition. Certainly, it will make the big drug companies very happy in having yet another long-term customer hooked on their products.

You can increase your thyroid function with a simple but vital supplement: iodine. Just how important is iodine?

Iodine is essential to a proper functioning thyroid. As we grow older, our thyroid starts slowing down. It just can't metabolize the iodine it needs as efficiently, and that means the hormone produced (also known as thyroid) goes down as well. There are many reasons why we might be iodine deficient, including:

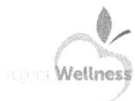
inadequate dietary intake and exposure to substances that displace iodine. Dietary intake is limited by the fact that iodine is a mineral and is not abundant in the food we eat. It can be found in very small quantities in seawater and soils close by but the further you get from the ocean the more limited the resource. Iodine exists naturally in most soils, and is taken up by plants, which in turn are eaten by humans and animals. Iodine is also fairly easily displaced from your body by toxins called toxic halides, which include fluoride, bromine, and chloride.

Fluoride is by far the worst culprit. Found in toothpaste and in your water supply, every time you take a shower, brush your teeth, or drink from the tap, your body gets a little exposure to fluoride leeching out good iodine.

Fluoride may have its place to prevent tooth decay, but clearly it affects our iodine stores. Due to these factors, 96% of all people tested are iodine deficient. The World Health Organization also concurs, estimating that 72% of the world's population is being affected by iodine deficiency. Over the last 30 years, iodine levels have dropped 50% in the U.S.A. alone.

The bottom line is that if there is not enough iodine in the thyroid gland, then it is impossible to have sufficient thyroid hormone of any type. The result is an underactive thyroid or hypothyroidism.

Here's where it gets a little tricky. There are two types of iodine necessary for optimal nutrition and thyroid function: iodine and iodide. The iodine supplements you normally find are made from kelp or seaweed lacking in iodide. Plus, the iodine supplements you'll see on the retail shelves are about 100 times weaker than they need to be. Iodine is present and used in every single cell in your body, including salivary glands, cerebrospinal fluid, and the brain, gastric mucosa, choroid plexus (part of the brain), breasts, ovaries, and eye ciliary bodies.

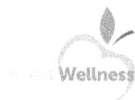

Most studies recommend a full 5 mg of iodine combined with a balanced amount of 7.5 mg of iodide for the optimal formulation for peak bio-availability along with selenium which enhances conversion of the inactive thyroid hormone T4 into the active thyroid hormone T3.

If you are currently taking a thyroid hormone like Synthroid, Levothroid, Levoxyl, or Armour, taking the iodine tablets will actually reduce the amount of your prescription dosage needed or may even eliminate it altogether.

If you are taking these prescription medications, please make sure you consult with your physician and take regular thyroid blood level tests.

My favorite form of iodine, Iodoral, can be purchased online at Amazon.com, Naturamart.com, and Life extension.com or at health food stores.

Iodoral is a tablet containing iodine and iodide as the potassium salt. To prevent gastric irritation, the iodine/iodide preparation is absorbed into a colloidal silica excipient. To eliminate the unpleasant taste of iodine, which is one of the major problems with liquid iodine supplement like Lugol's solution, the tablets are coated with a thin film of pharmaceutical glaze.

For adults, the recommended daily allowance is 150 micrograms, if you do not have symptoms of underactive thyroid function. Most of the human body's stores of iodine are located in the thyroid gland, which requires it for the synthesis of thyroid hormones.

Sometimes, patients tell me they can't take iodine because they are allergic. Allergic reactions to iodine usually stem from iodine-based contrast dyes injected to sharpen pictures in medical imaging studies, such as X-rays and CT scans. These reactions, typically, are mild and involve nausea, vomiting, itching, flushing, and hives.

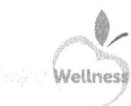

But in some cases, reactions can be quite severe (anaphylaxis) with swelling of the throat, difficulty breathing, profound low blood pressure, convulsions, and cardiac arrest. If you've experienced a severe reaction as a result of the dye used for an imaging study, make sure your physician and the radiologist supervising any future X-rays or scans are fully aware of your history.

A reaction to an iodine-based dye is not the same thing as an allergy to iodine because it generally doesn't stem from the same type of immune-system response as a true allergy. Having a reaction to an iodine-based contrast dye is also not the same as an allergy to seafood, which may be rich in iodine. If you're reacting to shellfish, the iodine it contains is unlikely to be responsible. It is more likely due to distinctive allergens found in these foods.

Most people who are allergic to shellfish react to certain proteins these foods contain, not to iodine. You can be allergic to all types of shellfish or only to one certain kind like mollusks (which include clams and oysters) or crustaceans (that include crabs and shrimp). Each of these two general types of shellfish contains different proteins. There is a small chance (about three percent) that if you're allergic to seafood, you'll have a reaction to contrast dye, but this is no more likely to happen than it is among people with other types of food allergies.

In general, if you reacted to an iodine-based contrast dye, you should be able to safely eat seafood and other foods high in iodine. If your reaction was to shellfish of some type, you are probably allergic to something other than iodine. And don't worry about your thyroid. Your body will get the trace amounts of iodine needed to make thyroid hormone from your diet.

So, now that you know you need iodine for conversion of inactive to the active form of thyroid, you need to understand the traditional approach is to use synthetic hormones like Synthroid / Levoxyl /

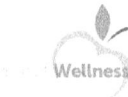
Levothroid (levothyroxine). These products only contain T4 hormone; they have no T3.

The common argument the physicians give is that the synthetic provides steady hormone levels. What the doctors tend to overlook is that the vast majority of people cannot convert the T4 to the active form of thyroid which is T3. This is easy to confirm by measuring the free hormone levels.

When one has low T3 levels, which are typical with synthetic hormone use, the brain does not work properly. It is important to use a preparation with T3 because T3 does 90% of the work of the thyroid in the body. So, one should use a combination of T4 and T3 which compensates for the inability to convert T4 to T3. Armour thyroid is desiccated thyroid and has both T3 and T4.

Another issue with Armour is it is most effective when dosed twice a day. The most common starting dose for patients with hypothyroidism is 90 mg, which is cut in half and taken after breakfast and the other half after dinner. Taking it after meals also helps to reduce volatility of the blood-level of T3. The TSH, Free T3 and Free T4 are then repeated in one month and the dose is adjusted.

Taking the Armour thyroid twice a day overcomes traditional medicine's major objection and resistance to using natural thyroid preparations – its variability in its blood-levels. Most doctors using Armour thyroid are not aware that Armour thyroid should be used twice daily and NOT once a day. The major reason is the T3 component has such a short half-life and needs to be taken twice daily to achieve consistent blood levels. The best way to adjust the thyroid hormone is to increase the dosage until the TSH falls below 0.4 and by measuring free T3 and free T4 levels.

The Free T3 and Free T4 are used to monitor the treatment. They should be above the median (middle) and below the upper end of

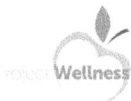

the laboratory normal reference range. The goal for healthy young adults would be to have numbers close to the upper part of the range, and for cardiac and/or elderly patients, the numbers should be in the middle of its range.

The Free T3 and Free T4 levels should be checked every month and the hormone therapy readjusted until the FT3 and FT4 levels are in the therapeutic range described. Once a therapeutic range is achieved the levels should be checked at least once a year. A small number of large, overweight, thyroid-resistant women may need 6-8 grains of Armour thyroid per day. If you experience nervousness, hot sweats, rapid weight loss, tremor, or clammy skin, then the dose should be decreased despite the lab level.

Some patients cannot tolerate Armour thyroid for various reasons and if this is the case you should consider taking compound natural hormone combinations.

Once or twice daily dosing one can then optimize both the T4 and T3 levels, with whatever thyroid preparation is required. This is not possible in most hypothyroid patients with T4 only preparations. Patients with congestive heart failure or severe lung problems may not be the best candidates for Armour because metabolic slowing effect of a low FT3 level can actually be life-saving. However, the vast majority of hypothyroid patients do not have this problem.

Armour thyroid provides the best results for the majority of patients. Armour thyroid not only contains T3 and T4, but it contains many other factors that facilitate the conversion of T4 to T3 including calcitonin, T1, T2, and many other chemicals. Armour Thyroid has been around for almost 100 years and has proven to be extremely safe and effective.

A number of factors can contribute to the inability to convert T4 to T3, including:

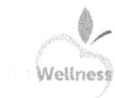

1. Deficiencies of zinc, selenium, iodine, and iron

2. Beta blockers, Dilantin, and certain other drugs

3. Alcohol, toxins, synthetic hormones, and pesticides

All patients with thyroid problems need to be properly evaluated for vitamin and mineral deficiencies. Just by correcting dietary insufficiencies, thyroid symptoms will usually improve. It is well known that adequate protein and fat is necessary to convert T4 to T3. Excessive iodine supplementation can aggravate some autoimmune thyroid conditions, so you have to be careful with iodine supplementation in these cases.

A deficiency of thyroid hormone can slow down metabolic actions in the body and cause weight gain. Consumption of soy protein can boost the body's natural secretion of thyroid hormone, thereby increasing the body's metabolic rate. Thyroid hormone also is necessary to drive glucose into the cells.

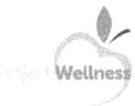
## What Your Lab Tests Mean

It is very important that you begin a roadmap of where you want to go. One of the first and foremost things that you will want to do is to understand where you are.

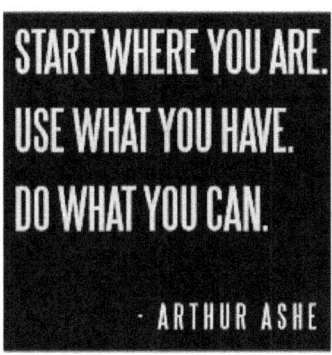

START WHERE YOU ARE.
USE WHAT YOU HAVE.
DO WHAT YOU CAN.

- ARTHUR ASHE

I have so many patients that come in for the first time and are completely clueless about anything to do with his/her health. The are on medications but don't know the names or doses. Sometimes I hear, "Oh, I'm on the little blue and white pill". There are literally hundreds if not thousands of little blue and white pills. And then they may be trying to treat a number like cholesterol, but have no idea what the goal number is and they just trust that the doctor knows what all mediations you are on and if there are side effects. The CDC (Centers for Disease Control) estimates that over 100,000 people in the United States die each year from prescription medications and these are taken as prescribed by the doctor. Do you want to be one of those statistics? That's incentive alone to know exactly what you are taking and what you are putting in your body and why. The first step in empowering yourself in your health and wellness is to understand what your basic lab values are and mean. You don't need a medical degree to understand these basics. Just like you have a GPS in your car. You don't need to understand how the electrical system works in your car or the computer system works in the GPS to get you

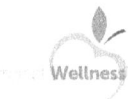

where you need to go, but you do need a basic understanding of how to plug in where you are and where you want to end up, right?

I wrote a book in medical school called "Healthy Ambitions-Tools for Taking Charge of Your Health Care", because I felt it was so important for people to be able to ask the right questions and get to the right answers. What follows is a basic lab test evaluation and explanation. These are the essential labs that we recommend in our wellness program and the basic interpretations. You will want to visit with your provider or coach to understand yours in more detail.

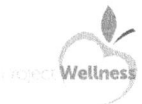

# What Your Lab Tests Mean

As you learn about how your body works and what these lab tests mean, we recommend that you keep a notebook, take notes and start your education in your personal individualized human body user's manual.

## Glucose:

This test should be performed with a 6-8 hour minimum fast. This is a measure of the sugar level in your blood. High values are associated with eating before the test, and diabetes. The normal range for a fasting glucose is 60 -99 mg/dl. According the 2003 ADA criteria, diabetes is diagnosed with a *fasting* plasma glucose of 126 or more. A precursor, Impaired Fasting Glucose (IFG) is defined as reading of fasting glucose levels of 100 - 125.

## Insulin:

Insulin is secreted by the pancreas in response to eating or elevated blood sugar. It is deficient in persons with type 1 diabetes, and present at insufficient levels in persons with type 2 diabetes. The natural evolution of type 2 diabetes causes insulin levels to fall from high levels to low levels over a course of years. Insulin levels vary widely from person to person depending upon an individuals insulin sensitivity (or conversely, their insulin resistance.) Insulin levels also vary widely according to when the last meal occurred. Insulin resistance is a risk factor for coronary disease.

This test should be performed with a 6-8 hour minimum fast. This is a measure of the insulin level in your blood. If you are truly fasting then insulin should be negligible or zero, because the sugar content in the blood should be low. Anything greater than 10 is considered pre-diabetes or insulin resistant. Greater than 5 may be considered to have insulin sensitivity issues.

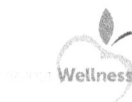

**My glucose is high or my insulin is elevated:**

[]Chromium 200 mcg with meals 2-3 times a day

[]Decrease Carbohydrates (sugar-simple and complex) to 25-30 grams/ meal

[]Order lab tests after changes for follow up in 3-6 months

[]Order **Glycohemoglobin** (Hemoglobin A1 or A1c, HbA1c) :
Glycohemoglobin measures the amount of glucose chemically attached to your red blood cells. Since blood cells live about 3 months, it tells us your average glucose for the last 6 - 8 weeks. A high level (greater than 6.5) suggests poor diabetes control

[]other: _____

# Waste products:

Blood Urea Nitrogen (BUN) is a waste product produced in the liver and excreted by the kidneys. High values may mean that the kidneys are not working as well as they should. BUN is also affected by high protein diets and/or strenuous exercise which raise levels, and by pregnancy which lowers it.

Creatinine is a waste product largely from muscle breakdown. High values, especially with high BUN levels, may indicate problems with the kidneys.

## Enzymes

AST, ALT, SGOT, SGPT, and GGT and Alkaline Phosphatase are abbreviations for proteins called enzymes which help all the chemical activities within cells to take place. Injury to cells release these enzymes into the blood. They are found in muscles, the liver and heart. Damage from medications (including over the counter) alcohol and a number of diseases are reflected in high values. Fatty liver, or those who have "Belly Fat" deposition to protect the organs and draw toxins away from them may have elevated levels.

## Proteins

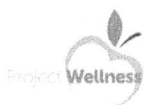

Total protein may be low with dietary intake deficiencies. Albumin and Globulin measure the amount and type of protein in your blood. They are a general index of overall health and nutrition. Globulin is the "antibody" protein important for fighting disease.

**My protein is low:**

[]Increase dietary protein (beans, vegetable protein etc.)

# Blood Fats

Total Cholesterol:

Cholesterol in itself is not all bad, in fact, our bodies need a certain amount of this substance to function properly. We need cholesterol for the brain to think and operate. We need cholesterol to make our sex steroid hormones.

There are three major kinds of cholesterol, High Density Lipoprotein (HDL) , Low Density Lipoprotein (LDL), and Very Low Density Lipoprotein (VLDL).

LDL Cholesterol is sometimes considered "bad cholesterol" because these cholesterol deposits could form in the arteries when inflammation is present at high levels. Values greater than 160 should be monitored and other inflammation risk factors addressed as well as life style changes recommended.

HDL cholesterol is a 'good cholesterol' as it protects against heart disease by helping remove excess cholesterol deposited in the arteries. High levels seem to be associated with low incidence of coronary heart disease.

Triglyceride is sugary-fat in the blood which, if elevated, has been associated with heart disease, especially if over 500 mg. High triglycerides are also

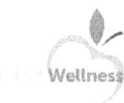 

associated with pancreatitis. Triglyceride levels over 150 mg/dl may be associated with problems other than heart disease.

## My cholesterol is high:

[]weight reduction, if overweight

[]regular aerobic exercise 30 min 3 times a week

[] Niacin (B-vitamin) supplement 500 mg/ day Slow release to reduce flushing

[]Fish oil 4000 mg/ day

[] decrease alcohol and sugar consumption—alcohol and sugar are not fats, but the body can convert them into fats then dump those fats into your blood stream

[]Increase Fiber to 25-30 grams/ day

## Inflammation /Cardiac Risk Markers

C Reactive Protein (CRP): This is a marker for inflammation. Traditionally it has been used to assess inflammation in response to infection. However we use a highly sensitive C Reactive Protein which is useful in predicting vascular disease, heart attack or stroke.

Homocysteine: Homocysteine is an amino acid that is normally found in small amounts in the blood. Higher levels are associated with increased risk of heart attack and other vascular diseases. Homocysteine levels may be high due to a deficiency of folate or Vitamin B12, due to heredity, older age, kidney disease, or certain medications. Men tend to have higher levels. Our lab normals are 4 - 15 micromole/l , but if you have had previous vascular disease we may recommend L-methyl-folate to reduce it below 10. You can reduce your homocysteine level by eating more green leafy vegetables and fortified grain products or cereals.

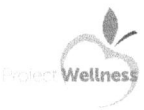

**My CRP and/ or homocysteine are elevated:**

[]L-methyl-folate 1000-2000 mg/ day

[]Omega-3 (fish oil) 2-6 grams/day

[]other: _____ anti-inflammatories (reservatrol, turmeric…), niacin, weight loss, quitting smoking, and exercise

## Minerals

Calcium is controlled in the blood by the parathyroid glands and the kidneys. Calcium is found mostly in bone and is important for proper blood clotting, nerve, and cell activity. An elevated calcium can be due to medications such as thiazide type diuretics, inherited disorders of calcium handling in the kidneys, or excess parathyroid gland activity or vitamin D. Low calcium can be due to certain metabolic disorders such as insufficient parathyroid hormone; or drugs like Fosamax or furosemide type diuretics. Calcium is bound to albumin in the blood, so a low albumin level will cause the total calcium level in the blood to drop. You doctor can easily determine if this is significant or not. Phosphorus is also largely stored in the bone. It is regulated by the kidneys, and high levels may be due to kidney disease. When low levels are seen with high calcium levels it suggests parathyroid disease, however there are other causes. A low phosphorus, in combination with a high calcium, may suggest an overactive parathyroid gland.

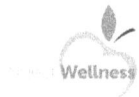

# Hormones

## Thyroid

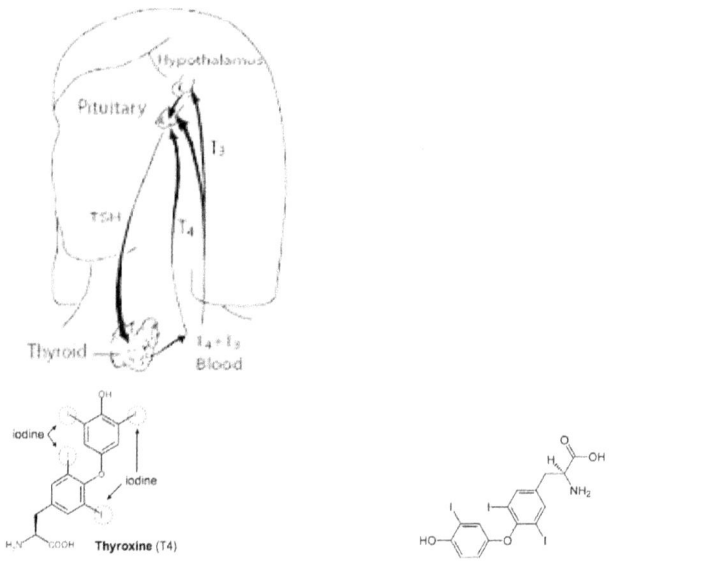

T4 (inactive or less active) ---peroxidase enzyme-----→ T3 (active)

There are 2 types of thyroid hormones easily measurable in the blood, thyroxine (T4) and tri-iodothyronine (T3).

Please be clear on which test you are looking at. We continue to see a tremendous amount of confusion among doctors, nurses, lab techs, and patients on which test is which. In particular, the "Total T3", "Free T3" and "T3 Uptake tests" are very confusing, and are not the same test.

**Free T3**: (FT3)  This test measures only the portion of thyroid hormone T3 that is "free", that is, not bound to carrier proteins. This should be optimized at the top of the range for maximum metabolism function.

**Thyroid Stimulating Hormone** (TSH) : This protein hormone is secreted by the pituitary gland and regulates the thyroid gland. A high level suggests your

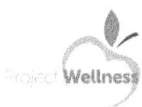

thyroid is underactive, and a low level suggests your thyroid is overactive. This test can vary by time of day, so a single abnormal measurement does not always mean there is a problem.

**Thyroid Antibodies**

Antimicrosomal Antibody is also known as Anti-Tissue Peroxidase (or Anti-TPO). It becomes elevated in autoimmune thyroid disease such as Hashimoto's Thyroiditis, or Graves' Disease. Anti-Thyroglobulin Antibody also becomes elevated in some cases of autoimmune thyroiditis. It tends to be positive more frequently in Graves' Disease than Hashimoto's. This test is also commonly used when following patients with thyroid cancer. In thyroid cancer patients, the Thyroglobulin test is used a marker for residual thyroid tissue. Elevated TPO and gluten sensitivity has strong correlations.

**My thyroid is abnormally:  []Low    []high**

[]I need thyroid support supplements (iodine, selenium, zinc…)

[]I need low dose thyroid supplementation with _____

[]I need to avoid all gluten products

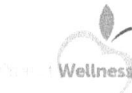

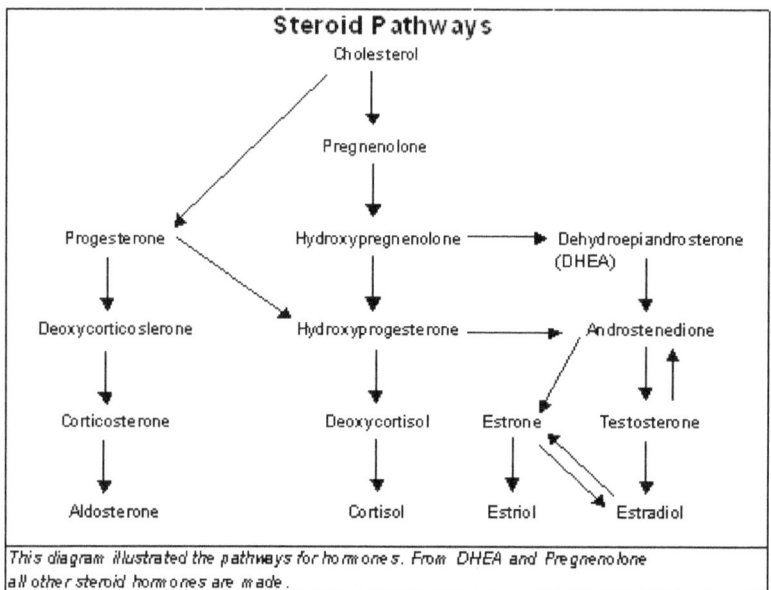

This diagram illustrated the pathways for hormones. From DHEA and Pregnenolone all other steroid hormones are made.

## Estrogens :

E1 (Estrone) =proliferative or problematic???

E2 (Estradiol) =neutral best for hot flashes

E3 (Estriol) =protective

In women the estrogens vary according to their age, and whether they are having normal menstrual cycles. Hormone levels are also changed when taking birth control pills or estrogen replacement.

**Testosterone** : This is the male sex hormone, however both men and women have detectable testosterone levels. In men the major source is the testicles, in women the ovaries. In men, low levels of testosterone can indicate reduced testicular function, or 'male hypogonadism'. This can be due to disease, aging, or damage to the testicles, 'testicular or primary hypogonadism'. It may also be due to inadequate function of the pituitary gland or hypothalamus 'secondary hypogonadism' from diseases that affect the

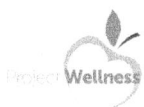

pituitary or adrenal issues. High testosterone can occur from testosterone injections, testosterone receptor defects, or testosterone secreting tumors.

In women, high testosterone levels can occur because of production from either the ovaries (like PCOS) or adrenal glands. Adrenal hormones such as DHEA can be converted in to testosterone.

**Progesterone:**

The yin to the yang of estrogen in both men and women. Must be in proper balance to promote mood, sleep and fluid balance.

## My hormones are out of balance:

[]I need hormone supplementation for __ months  with

_____

[]I need supplements _____

[]I need cycled progesterone taken days 12-21 of menstrual cycle

## Complete Blood Count (CBC)

The CBC typically has several parameters that are created from an automated cell counter. These are the most relevant:

**White Blood Count (WBC)** is the number of white cells. High WBC can be a sign of infection. WBC is also increased in certain types of leukemia. Low white counts can be a sign of bone marrow diseases or an enlarged spleen.

**Hemoglobin (Hgb) and Hematocrit (Hct)** : The hemoglobin is the amount of oxygen carrying protein contained within the red blood cells. The hematocrit is the percentage of the blood volume occupied by red blood cells. In most labs the Hgb is actually measured, while the Hct is computed using the RBC

161

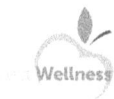
measurement and the MCV measurement. Thus purists prefer to use the Hgb measurement as more reliable. Low Hgb or Hct suggest an anemia. Anemia can be due to nutritional deficiencies, blood loss, destruction of blood cells internally, or failure to produce blood in the bone marrow. High Hgb can occur due to lung disease, living at high altitude, or excessive bone marrow production of blood cells.

**Mean Corpuscular Volume (MCV)** - This helps diagnose a cause of an anemia. Low values suggest iron deficiency, high values suggest either deficiencies of B12 or Folate, ineffective production in the bone marrow, or recent blood loss with replacement by newer (and larger) cells from the bone marrow.

**Platelet Count (PLT)** : This is the number of cells that plug up holes in your blood vessels and prevent bleeding. High values can occur with bleeding, cigarette smoking or excess production by the bone marrow. Low values can occur from premature destruction states such as Immune Thrombocytopenia (ITP), acute blood loss, drug effects (such as heparin), infections with sepsis, entrapment of platelets in an enlarged spleen, or bone marrow failure from diseases such as myelofibrosis or leukemia. Low platelets also can occur from clumping of the platelets in a lavender colored tube. You may need to repeat the test with a green top tube in that case.

# B12
Crucial supplement to metabolism.

[]Levels are low, recommend: []B12 injections 1 / week for ____weeks
[] Supplements: _____

# Iron

May be a cause of restless leg syndrome, fatigue and sleep or metabolic issues.

[]Levels are low, recommend: []Elemental iron ____ mg daily
[] Supplements: _____

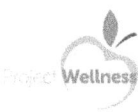

## Vitamin D
[]Levels are low, recommend:   []Vitamin D 50000 IU daily   []10000 IU daily
[] Supplements: _____

## Other: _____
_____
_____

## Questions to ask my provider or coach:
    1. _____
    2. _____
    3. _____
    4. _____
    5. _____

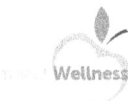

## Pharmaceuticals… Is it your choice???

# Blood Pressure Medication
*Your decision…Your Choice*

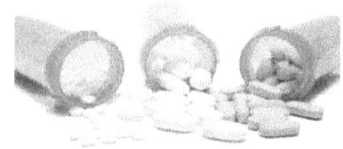

Deciding to take or to continue taking blood pressure medication can be a daunting decision. Is it safe? Does the benefit outweigh the risk? How do you know?

Are blood pressure medications bad?

The answer is no! The problem is that fear drives many well meaning physicians to scare patients into taking them even when possibly not appropriate. They can cause many side effects. While they lower blood pressure, the bigger concern is that they are just masking the symptoms of a bigger problem. The main problem with blood pressure medications is this: You don't want to choose a medication to lower a blood pressure number. To me, that's bad medicine and I'll tell you why.

Blood pressure medication drugs can have horrific side effects:

- Low blood pressure (feeling tired and light headed, possibly falling)
- Memory issues: pre-Alzheimer's condition (people literally forget who they are or act in unsafe ways).

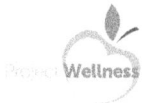

- Difficulty with vision
- Liver problems, kidney problems, polyneuropathy (nerve issues)
- Hormone imbalance
- And many more…

How These Drugs Work

First of all, while these medications lower your numbers, they do nothing to treat the underlying cause. There are many blood pressure medications and they work in many different ways.  Usually to lower your sodium (salt in the blood) and therefore can make you crave more salt.

Why do doctors prescribe them?

Mostly because it is easy to just prescribe a pill.  It's fast and gets the patient out the door and effective to some degree, but ultimately it's because they don't have the time to educate you about natural ways to do this.  When I used to treat pregnant women, we didn't use many blood pressure mediations because we knew it was harmful to the baby.  You know what we used?  Dietary changes and MAGNESIUM.

When to Take Blood Pressure Drugs

So, when do you take a blood pressure drug?  When your levels are dangerously high (220/120) is what we refer to as "stroke levels.  If you have time to make lifestyle changes this is the preferred route.  It is also very important to understand the underlying cause.

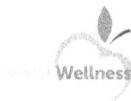

What are the underlying causes?

- age – the risk of developing high blood pressure increases as you get older, less elasticity of the blood vessels from inflammation
- genetics- a family history of high blood pressure (the condition seems to run in families)
- being of African or Caribbean origin
- a high amount of salt in your food
- a lack of exercise
- being overweight or obese
- smoking
- drinking large amounts of alcohol
- kidney disease
- diabetes
- narrowing of the arteries (large blood vessels) supplying the kidneys
- hormonal conditions
- conditions that affect the body's tissue, such as lupus
- oral contraceptive pill
- painkillers known as nonsteroidal anti-inflammatory drugs (NSAIDs), such as ibuprofen
- recreational drugs, such as cocaine, amphetamines and crystal methamphetamine
- herbal remedies, such as herbal supplements

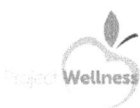

Big Pharmacies are busy raking in over $31 billion annually by selling blood pressure drugs with terrible side effects to unknowing victims, their success is putting the American public's health at risk.

References and further reading to make an informed decision

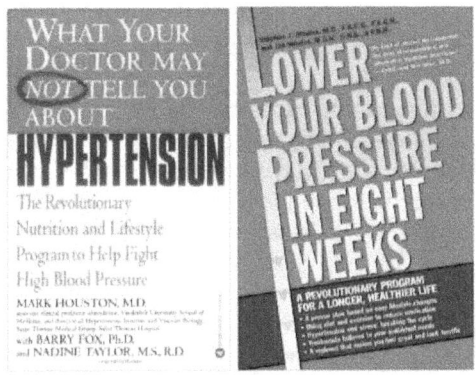

http://www.drsinatra.com/

Natural ways to manage inflammation and lower blood pressure

Fish oil (Omega-3)
Niacin
Co-Q-10
Vitamin K
Reservatrol and Tumeric
B-Vitamins (Methy-B12 and Methyl-Folate)
Magnesium
Fiber
Exercise
Hormone balance

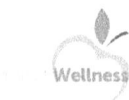

# Magnesium

The mineral magnesium plays several key roles in the body, including the regulation of blood pressure. People who eat diets rich in this nutrient along with others such as potassium tend to have lower blood pressure compared to people whose diets lack adequate levels

## Dosage Guidelines

The suggested daily dosage for magnesium hinges on gender. The UMMC notes a dosage range of 270 mg to 400 mg for men and 280 mg to 300 mg for women. Dr. Michael T. Murray, an expert on the role of nutrition in health, recommends taking 150 mg to 250 mg three to four times a day to treat hypertension. This greatly exceeds the dosages recommended to ensure adequate intake and promote general health. Often, you might require larger doses of a vitamin or mineral to achieve a medicinal effect. Work with your doctor in these instances since high amounts of natural substances can carry the risk for adverse reactions much like drugs can.

## Side Effects and Safety Concerns

If you have heart or kidney disease, do not supplement with magnesium without your doctor's supervision. Common side effects include diarrhea and stomach upset. If you already have low stores of calcium, magnesium supplementation could lead to a calcium deficiency because these nutrients compete for absorption. Talk to your doctor about the need for a calcium supplement while using magnesium. When taken at the suggested dosages, the use of supplements appears safe.

## Medication Interactions

Magnesium could decrease the effectiveness of several medications, including the antibiotics ciprofloxacin, moxifloxacin, tetracycline, doxycycline and minocycline and the osteoporosis medications tiludronate and alendronate. To avoid interactions, take magnesium supplements either one hour prior to taking these drugs or two hours after. If you take medications to manage your blood pressure, the use of supplements that exert similar effects could necessitate dosage adjustments to compensate for actions of magnesium. Only your doctor

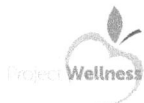

can safely make these determinations. Do not alter your treatments on your own.

Monitoring your blood pressure

First buy a cuff to have at home.

If you've been diagnosed with high blood pressure (a systolic pressure — the top number — of 140 or above or a diastolic pressure — the bottom number — of 90 or above), you might be worried about taking medication to bring your numbers down.

Lifestyle plays an important role in treating your high blood pressure. If you successfully control your blood pressure with a healthy lifestyle, you may avoid, delay or reduce the need for medication.

Here are 10 lifestyle changes you can make to lower your blood pressure and keep it down.

### 1. Lose extra pounds and watch your waistline

Blood pressure often increases as weight increases. Losing just 10 pounds (4.5 kilograms) can help reduce your blood pressure. In general, the more weight you lose, the lower your blood pressure. Losing weight also makes any blood pressure medications you're taking more effective. You and your doctor can determine your target weight and the best way to achieve it.

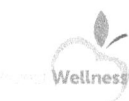

Besides shedding pounds, you should also keep an eye on your waistline. Carrying too much weight around your waist can put you at greater risk of high blood pressure. In general:

- Men are at risk if their waist measurement is greater than 40 inches (102 centimeters, or cm).

- Women are at risk if their waist measurement is greater than 35 inches (89 cm).

### 2. Exercise regularly

Regular physical activity — at least 30 to 60 minutes most days of the week — can lower your blood pressure by 4 to 9 millimeters of mercury (mm Hg). And it doesn't take long to see a difference. If you haven't been active, increasing your exercise level can lower your blood pressure within just a few weeks.

If you have prehypertension — systolic pressure between 120 and 139 or diastolic pressure between 80 and 89 — exercise can help you avoid developing full-blown hypertension. If you already have hypertension, regular physical activity can bring your blood pressure down to safer levels.

Talk to your doctor about developing an exercise program. Your doctor can help determine whether you need any exercise restrictions. Even moderate activity for 10 minutes at a time, such as walking and light strength training, can help.

But avoid being a "weekend warrior." Trying to squeeze all your exercise in on the weekends to make up for weekday

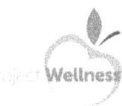

inactivity isn't a good strategy. Those sudden bursts of activity could actually be risky.

### 3. Eat a healthy diet

Eating a diet that is rich in vegetables and avoiding dairy products can lower your blood pressure by up to 14 mm Hg. This eating plan is known as the Dietary Approaches to Stop Hypertension (DASH) diet.

It isn't easy to change your eating habits, but with these tips, you can adopt a healthy diet:

- **Keep a food diary.** Writing down what you eat, even for just a week, can shed surprising light on your true eating habits. Monitor what you eat, how much, when and why.

- **Consider boosting potassium.** Potassium can lessen the effects of sodium on blood pressure. The best source of potassium is food, such as fruits and vegetables, rather than supplements. Talk to your doctor about the potassium level that's best for you.

- **Be a smart shopper.** Make a shopping list before heading to the supermarket to avoid picking up junk food. Read food labels when you shop and stick to your healthy-eating plan when you're dining out, too.

- **Cut yourself some slack.** Although the DASH diet is a lifelong eating guide, it doesn't mean you have to cut out all of the foods you love. It's OK to treat yourself occasionally to foods you wouldn't find on a DASH diet menu, such as a candy bar or mashed potatoes with gravy.

4. Reduce sodium in your diet

Even a small reduction in the sodium in your diet can reduce blood pressure by 2 to 8 mm Hg. The recommendations for reducing sodium are:

- Limit sodium to 2,300 milligrams (mg) a day or less.

- A lower sodium level — 1,500 mg a day or less — is appropriate for people 51 years of age or older, and individuals of any age who are African-American or who have high blood pressure, diabetes or chronic kidney disease.

To decrease sodium in your diet, consider these tips:

- **Track how much salt is in your diet.** Keep a food diary to estimate how much sodium is in what you eat and drink each day.

- **Read food labels.** If possible, choose low-sodium alternatives of the foods and beverages you normally buy.

- **Eat fewer processed foods.** Potato chips, frozen dinners, bacon and processed lunch meats are high in sodium.

- **Don't add salt.** Just 1 level teaspoon of salt has 2,300 mg of sodium. Use herbs or spices, rather than salt, to add more flavor to your foods.

- **Ease into it.** If you don't feel like you can drastically reduce the sodium in your diet suddenly, cut back gradually. Your palate will adjust over time.

5. Limit the amount of alcohol you drink

Alcohol can be both good and bad for your health. In small amounts, it can potentially lower your blood pressure by 2 to 4 mm Hg. But that protective effect is lost if you drink too

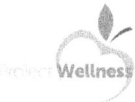

much alcohol — generally more than one drink a day for women and men older than age 65, or more than two a day for men age 65 and younger. Also, if you don't normally drink alcohol, you shouldn't start drinking as a way to lower your blood pressure. There's more potential harm than benefit to drinking alcohol.

If you drink more than moderate amounts of it, alcohol can actually raise blood pressure by several points. It can also reduce the effectiveness of high blood pressure medications.

- **Track your drinking patterns.** Along with your food diary, keep an alcohol diary to track your true drinking patterns. One drink equals 12 ounces (355 milliliters, or mL) of beer, 5 ounces of wine (148 mL) or 1.5 ounces of 80-proof liquor (45 mL). If you're drinking more than the suggested amounts, cut back.

- **Consider tapering off.** If you're a heavy drinker, suddenly eliminating all alcohol can actually trigger severe high blood pressure for several days. So when you stop drinking, do it with the supervision of your doctor or taper off slowly, over one to two weeks.

- **Don't binge.** Binge drinking — having four or more drinks in a row — can cause large and sudden increases in blood pressure, in addition to other health problems.

6.  **To Control High Blood Pressure, Be Careful with synthetic Hormone Replacement Therapy (HRT):** In 2004, results were published from the Women's Health Initiative, a study including women taking Premarin. The women taking this pharmaceutical form of estrogen, (made from the urine of pregnant mares), were

173

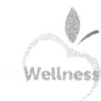

observed to have "skyrocketing" blood pressure levels. But
Premarin is not the only HRT that causes high blood pressure.

> Dr. Sinatra has noted that Provera, another HRT mainstay,
> drove up blood pressure in the women he treated, many of
> whom were no longer hypertensive once they discontinued the
> drug.
>
> What we're learning is that to control high blood pressure,
> individually tailored bio-identical hormone therapy from more
> natural plant and synthetic sources are better for women.
> Combining estradiole, estriol, estrone, testosterone, and
> progesterone may soften those arterial walls that can stiffen
> with age, and may even intercept elevating blood pressure.  So
> please consider this approach if you are on the traditional HRT
> medications, especially if you're trying to control high blood
> pressure.

7.  **Watch the Painkillers:** A report from the Harvard School of
    Medicine's ongoing Nurses Health Study, published in the
    September 2005 issue of *Hypertension*, concluded that women
    are at increased risk for high blood pressure if they take daily
    doses of non-aspirin painkillers such as extra-strength
    acetaminophen and ibuprofen.

    If you take painkillers regularly and are trying to control high
    blood pressure, please ask your doctor for safer
    recommendations. What we use at our house—and it works
    well for various muscle aches and pains—is Traumeel, a
    homeopathic remedy you can find in health food stores.
    Traumeel is available in both a topical cream and a tablet that
    you place under your tongue.

8.  **Eat More Garlic:**  An Australian review of 11 studies in
    which hypertensive patients were randomly given a garlic
    supplement or placebo, found that garlic can lower blood
    pressure as effectively as some drugs. On average, the mega-
    analysis turned up blood pressure reductions of 8.4 systolic
    points, and 7.3 diastolic points. The higher a patient's blood
    pressure was at the beginning, the more it was lowered by
    taking garlic.

174

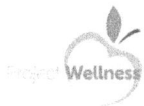

To control high blood pressure, I recommend four cloves of raw garlic (about four grams) daily to achieve a noticeable blood pressure lowering effect. You could also toss crushed garlic into food for the last few minutes of cooking, but anything more than lightly warming it will destroy its medicinal properties to control high blood pressure.

9. **De-Stress—It's a Surefire Way to Control High Blood Pressure:** Stress is a major mitigating factor when it comes to your blood pressure, so be aware of the psychological pressures you're juggling. Overachieving and time urgency are all-too common "normals" for women. We juggle multiple roles as breadwinner, wife, daughter, mother, and friend that often involve nurturing others at our own expense if we don't refuel.

   Some good ways to de-stress and control high blood pressure include meditation, relaxation, imagery, yoga, prayer, Tai Chi, exercise, reading, listening to calming music, or playing with children and friends into your daily life.

   Also remember that not all venting is "complaining." Talking with someone you trust about the stresses in your life, benefits your wellbeing—and helps you control high blood pressure.

Lastly, remember to stay positive! No one is sentenced to a life of high blood pressure because of her DNA. It's not our destiny! Our blood pressure reading is only a number, and it's one we can lower with our own conscientious lifestyle changes, and medication if needed.

*2 grams/2000mg*

**Did you know? (those with high blood pressure should consume less than 2000 mg or 2 grams a day)**

*"But, I don't use salt!" I hear this all the time.   Consider this….*

*Pancakes with syrup contains 1,104 mg of salt*

*Low fat cottage cheese 1 cup has 918 mg*

*1 cup of Tuna Salad has 824 mg*

*Diet Soda has 70 mg*

The average intake of salt (sodium chloride) in the U.S. is approximately 9 grams per day, which contains 150 mmol, or 3.5 grams, of sodium per day. Reductions in the daily sodium intake to 100 mmol (2.3 grams), and then to 50 mmol (1.2 grams), lead to sequential reductions in blood pressure. When dietary salt restriction is combined with the DASH diet, an even greater reduction in blood pressure occurs at each level of sodium intake. The studies have indicated that the groups who have the best response to this combined approach are people older than 45 years, patients with hypertension, and African-Americans. Importantly, it is also thought that younger people with normal blood pressures who follow these combined dietary guidelines may develop less hypertension, as they get older.

Ways to taste good without salt:
Use juice or wine or flavored vinegars (you can stir fry veggies and meat in apple juice, white grape juice, wine etc.  Go heavy on other seasonings such as pepper, basil, oregano, fresh tomatoes, onions, garlic and fresh lemon or thyme Mint and basil work well for steak or meat

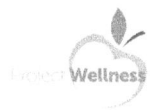

Pork does well with chili powder and cumin
Chicken does well with garlic and lemon and thyme

ALWAYS check labels, one brand may have different amounts than other brands, you never know until you look.

### Reading a Food Label for Sodium Content

1. Begin by reviewing the serving size and sodium content information. See the shaded areas on the sample label to the right.

   The serving size for the food on this label is 5 oz. (ounces). The sodium content for that serving is 440 mg.

2. If you eat the same sized serving as the one listed on the label, then you are eating the amount of sodium that is listed.

   But if the amount you actually eat is either larger or smaller, the amount of sodium you will be eating will also be larger or smaller.

   For example, if you eat a double portion of the food shown above, you will also be eating twice as much sodium as listed on the label. A 10 oz. serving of the food above would contain 880 mg of sodium.

# Nutrition Facts

Serving Size 5 oz
Servings Per Container 4

**Amount Per Serving**

**Calories** 90      Calories from Fat 30

|  | % Daily Value* |
|---|---|
| **Total Fat** 3g | 5% |
| Saturated Fat 0g | 0% |
| **Cholesterol** 0mg | 0% |
| **Sodium** 440mg | 19% |
| **Total Carbohydrate** 13g | 4% |
| Dietary Fiber 3g | 4% |
| Sugars 3g | |
| **Protein** 3g | |

| Vitamin A | 80% | • | Vitamin C | 60% |
|---|---|---|---|---|
| Calcium | 4% | • | Iron | 4% |

\* Percent Daily Values are based on a 2,000 calorie diet. Your daily values may be higher or depending on your calorie needs:

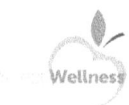
Wellness

# Cholesterol Medication
*Your decision…Your Choice*

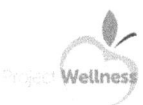
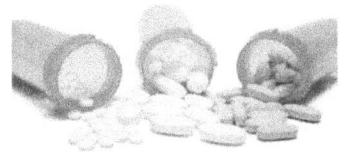

Deciding to take or to continue taking Cholesterol medication can be a daunting decision. Is it safe? Does the benefit outweigh the risk? How do you know?

## Are Statin Drug's bad?

The answer is no! The problem is that fear drives many well meaning physicians to scare patients into taking them even when possibly not appropriate. Statins are a blessing and a curse, because they do incredibly good things, but they can do bad things. The problem with a statin is this: You don't want to choose a statin to lower a cholesterol number. To me, that's bad medicine and I'll tell you why.

Statin drugs can have horrific side effects:

- Weakness of the limbs
- Memory issues: pre-Alzheimer's condition (people literally forget who they are or act in unsafe ways).
- Difficulty with vision
- Liver problems, kidney problems, polyneuropathy (nerve issues)
- Hormone imbalance

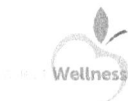
- And many more…

## How Statin Drugs Work

First of all, statin drugs happen to lower cholesterol numbers, but the way they really work is they're anti-inflammatory agents-and we know that inflammation is the *cause* of coronary artery disease. So, if you take an anti-inflammatory like a statin drug, could you do your vessel some good? Yes, you could. The other thing a statin does: It changes the shape of red blood cells. In other words, we use that term, "blood rheology," it has an effect on blood aggregation where it can literally make the blood cells less sticky. So, statin drugs work in two ways. They're potent anti-inflammatory agents and they make the blood less viscous.  But Omega-3 Fish oil can do the same thing without the bad side effects.

## Who Should Use Statin Drugs

So, would I use them in a coronary population with advanced coronary disease? Of course I would. But I'm specific. I especially like statin drugs in men, ages between 50 and 75. Why not above 75? Well, I'll tell you. In patients over 75, I don't get as much bang for my buck. In other words, I don't really see the usefulness of a statin for elderly people because I'm more afraid of CNS [central nervous system] effects and memory effects. And remember, whenever I choose to use a statin drug, I give every one of my patients,

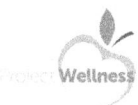

either male or female, at least 200 milligrams of CoQ10, because the side effects of statin drugs is that they're marvelous cholesterol killers because they intercept about 20 different biochemical pathways; one of those pathways is for CoQ10. So whenever you take a statin drug, you must, you must give yourself CoQ10 and I like at least 200 milligrams.

Now, what other population do we use statin drugs in? Well, I do use them in women, but only in women with advanced coronary artery disease, especially diabetic women, women with inflammatory mediators such as high C-reactive protein, women who are progressing downhill and they're getting more and more symptomatic-I use a statin drug. But in general I have not been as impressed with women with a statin drug as I am with middle age men.

Where else would I use a statin drug? Well, in anybody with advanced heart disease, whether a stent or angioplasty, heart attack, anybody with a high calcium score, even a calcium score over 200, I would use a statin drug, but not to lower cholesterol, folks. I use a statin drug to have an impact on the blood thinning, the blood rheology, the blood viscosity, and as an anti-inflammatory. So, if I had a male, for example, with a very low HDL and coronary calcium, I would use a low dose statin drug, because a low HDL makes the

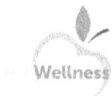

blood more viscous, it makes the blood more like red ketchup and that's the reason why a male with a low HDL is more prone to heart disease. So, I would use a statin drug in that situation, but, again, I don't treat numbers. One of the more common consults I saw in my office was a woman who would come in with a cholesterol of 280 and an HDL of 100 and her doctor would put her on a statin drug. To me, that's bad medicine. Why? Because, again, statin drugs deplete CoQ10 and CoQ10 is one of the most important nutrients to protect your immune system.

## When to Take Statin Drugs

So, when do you take a statin drug? To summarize, if you have advanced coronary disease, you're a middle age male, you have inflammatory mediators, you have coronary calcification, you're diabetic, and if you're a woman, where the coronary artery disease is getting out of control; those are the populations that would use statin drugs. To treat your cholesterol? No, I want to lifestyle interventions first.

## Cholesterol is the precursor to all your sex steroid hormones

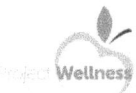
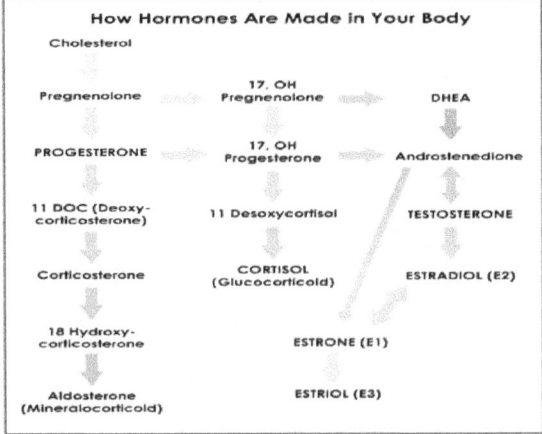

How Hormones Are Made In Your Body

Cholesterol

Pregnenolone → 17, OH Pregnenolone → DHEA

PROGESTERONE → 17, OH Progesterone → Androstenedione

11 DOC (Deoxy-corticosterone)   11 Desoxycortisol   TESTOSTERONE

Corticosterone   CORTISOL (Glucocorticoid)   ESTRADIOL (E2)

18 Hydroxy-corticosterone   ESTRONE (E1)

Aldosterone (Mineralocorticoid)   ESTRIOL (E3)

The decision must be an informed one and based on the whole patient not just a number or to "prevent a heart attack or stroke"

- The hypothetical link between high levels of total cholesterol and heart disease has NEVER been proven. It's a diagnosis conjured up to serve drug companies who want to sell cholesterol-lowering statin drugs.

- Cholesterol levels are a poor predictor of heart attacks. Only about 50% of heart attack victims have high cholesterol levels, and 50% of people who have high cholesterol do not have heart disease.

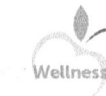
- Recent studies suggest statin drugs are associated with a higher risk of diabetes, which is a major risk factor for heart disease.

Big Pharmacies are busy raking in over $31 billion annually by selling high-cholesterol drugs with terrible side effects to unknowing victims, their success is putting the American public's health at risk.

Labs that should be checked for a comprehensive risk factor evaluation:

-CRP (inflammation marker)
-Homocysteine
-Insulin
-Hormones
-Thyroid

Chronic inflammation is a major predictor of coronary artery disease. Studies show elevated levels of CRP (inflammation) puts you at twice the risk of dying from cardiovascular-related problems as those with high cholesterol. Your doctor can order a CRP blood test, and while results may vary by lab you generally want a reading below 1.0.

References and further reading to make an informed decision

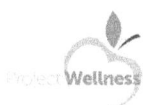

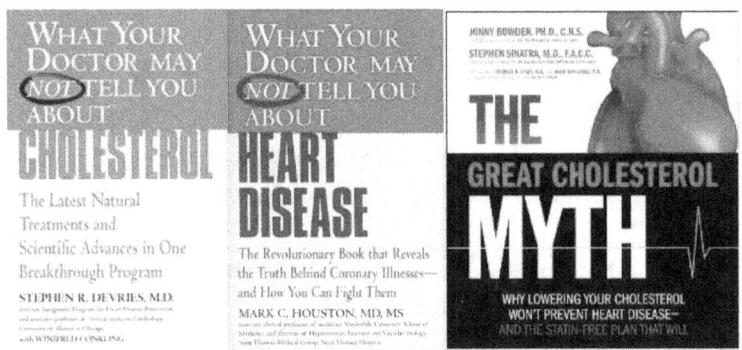

http://www.drsinatra.com/the-great-cholesterol-myth

Natural ways to manage inflammation and lower cholesterol

Fish oil (Omega-3)
Niacin
Co-Q-10
Vitamin K
Reservatrol and Tumeric
B-Vitamins (Methy-B12 and Methyl-Folate)
Magnesium
Fiber
Exercise
Hormone balance

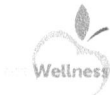
Wellness

# Project Stress

Are you stressed out? You are not alone. Seven out of ten adults in the U.S. say that they experience stress or anxiety on a regular basis. This stress can interfere with your life and daily function.

What is stress? The definition of stress, as my husband, the guru of stress, describes it, is the brain and body's (physical, chemical and neuro-hormonal) reaction to a perceived internal or external threat.

Stress is a good thing. It motivates us and is a natural response of protection. The problem is when stress is prolonged, overwhelming, and/or unpredictable. Stress can be long-term or short-term.

I like to break down stress into time frames.

Is this a
5-minute stress
5-hour stress
5-day stress
5-month stress
or
5-year stress?

There are three main kinds of stress that humans have to balance on a daily basis:
1. Physical stress: this can be from injury/trauma, over exercising, inflammation/arthritis in the body, etc.
2. Chemical stress: this is from toxins in the environment, alcohol, cigarettes, illegal drugs, medications, environmental pollutants, preservatives, etc.
3. Emotional stress: this is usually in the form of disunity in relationships, financial burdens, safety issues, work anxiety, and feeling overwhelmed.

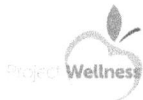

My main focus now is to help you with dealing with "Emotional Stress." Emotional stress is one of the biggest challenges that you will face in life.

Where do you start? You feel overwhelmed. Maybe you are having anxiety or panic attacks. You feel that life is too hard and maybe not even worth living at times. You can't get any relief. Work is stressful, then you come home and the family is stressing you out. You can't relax. You feel like you can't give anyone the love and attention you need because you have nothing left over to give. When you are at work, you feel like you should be at home. When you are home, you feel like you should be at work. Sleep is fractured and thoughts racing. How do you stop the madness?

The first thing you need to do is just notice how you are feeling. Recognize your emotions. You can't heal the stress without first recognizing it. Sometimes we just keep busy and ignore how we are feeling and that can be helpful at times, but if you really want to start reducing stress in your life and feel emotionally healthy, you will need a few steps to follow:

1. Get help for physical and chemical stress and deal with addictions
2. Get healthy physically, exercise, take supplements that help with stress, and focus on nutrition and learn to listen to what your body needs
3. Recognize how you feel and honor it
4. Spend some time thinking about what you want
5. Focus on what you want
6. Focus on gratitude for what you currently have
7. Learn to slow down (I won't scare you off by calling this meditation just yet)
8. Reframe
9. Learn to separate "distorted reality" from "real reality"

10. Learn the process of inquiry
11. Learn healthy boundaries
12. Have FUN!

1. Let's start with addictions:

How to be free of your addictions and anxiety, FOREVER!

Anxiety is just an inner state of unrest that is asking for you to soothe it. Addictions are attempts to self-soothe.

Are you addicted? To anything? To cigarettes, food, sugar, sex, shopping, drugs, a person (unhealthy relationship)?

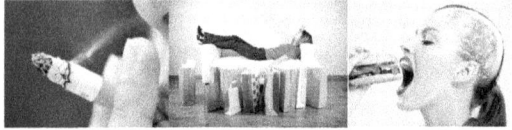

Here are some effective steps to breaking your addiction:

**Take supplements that decrease anxiety and calm pathways in the brain for dopamine or the addiction brain chemical:**
Niacin see internet references on creator of Alcoholics Anonymous, Bill Wilson
Magnesium – calms the nerves
Fish oil – anti-inflammatory that calms and improves brain nerve connectivity
N-acetylcysteine – calms neurotransmitters/brain chemicals
Methyl Folate – clears toxins and unhealthy unbalanced hormones from the liver and helps with depression, which can trigger addictive self-soothing behaviors
Methyl B12 – necessary to prevent depression, fatigue, anxiety, and addiction at the cellular/DNA level

Focus on getting healthy
Get a blood test for:
Mineral and vitamin nutritional levels

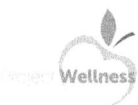

Hormone levels (including insulin, and thyroid as well as ovarian and testicular/adrenal)
Food sensitivities

Start an exercise routine: Walking is great to clear the mind, dancing is enjoyable

Focus on eating healthy

When you feel the addictive thought creep in, remember you don't have to chase every thought like a dog chases a scent in the air. When you feel anxious, ask yourself if what you know about a situation is true. Can you absolutely know that it is true?
Make a new story around your anxious thought. Creative people are more creative in their ability to form stories around events. Creative people often exaggerate negative aspects as they can be more exciting and "dramatic." Choose to be more boring in your negative storytelling or enhancements. Choose to err on the side of giving people the benefit of the doubt.

It is the story that tortures you. Obsessive thoughts play out in a negative way.
Focus on what you want to create. Obsess about what you want, but only on the positive outcome. Use your creativity to create an elaborate story of something beautiful and welcome in your life.

Addictions are just an attempt to short-circuit your brain, and therefore, the stories or obsessive thinking. They are merely a temporary distraction and keep you from having to do the real work of identifying what stresses you and understanding the power it has over you.

Create a new story

"How do I do this?" You might ask. The good news is the more creative you are, the better you will be at this process. The more terrified and crippled you are by your old stories just means that you are a delicious creator of stories. You should be being paid millions of dollars for your stories that you tell yourself and BELIEVE! We will discuss how to dismantle old stories, but for now, if you are a great story creator you need to focus on just creating new stories that serve you instead of ones that don't serve you.

First, you need to BREATHE. This sounds simple and everyone is always saying that you need to meditate. Meditation is only stopping the brain for a few minutes, so yes this is a version of meditation. Close your eyes and roll them up into your head as if you were looking into your mind. Breathe from your feet like you were sucking the breath up into a tall vacuum cleaner, or imagine the wave of an ocean washing up over you and back down. Do this 5 slow times.

Become aware of your surroundings… Become aware of your body… Begin to ask yourself…
> Am I hungry?
> Am I hot or cold?
> Am I tense or nervous?
> Am I tired?

If you are hungry, as simple as it sounds, then EAT! If you are cold, put on a jacket or comfy sweater, turn up the heat or turn on the AC, or just splash some cold water on your face. If you are tense, take a walk, scream in a pillow, do something to pattern-interrupt your brain, like standing on your head, tapping your chest, or spinning around in a circle. If you are tired, take a nap or just close your eyes and embrace the tiredness.

Address your physical issues… Ask yourself these questons… Do I have physical pain? Do I have gas? Headache? Stiffness? Thank your body for being able to process food, think for you, and move. Be kind to it and acknowledge that you have not always

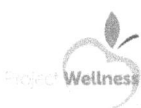

been kind to it. Find a more comfortable position, go to the bathroom, or take a hot bath or shower.

When you have addressed all your physical needs, then ask yourself how you are feeling emotionally.

What words come to mind? Anxious, sad, hurt, confused, angry…

Own the feeling!

I am _____(sad, anxious, hurt, scared…), because _____. It's okay if you don't know why right away. If you don't know the "because," then ask yourself,
"What am I afraid will happen to me?"

Ask where it is really coming from. Old hurts. Sit with the feeling for a few minutes and try to identify the trigger. The mind will produce one of our old stories pretty quickly.

Embrace your old story. Wow, you are a wonderful creator of stories. Give yourself a big hug for being so creative. So creative and convincing that you actually have yourself believing it! Imagine presenting yourself an Emmy award for the script and yourself as an actor for playing it out so perfectly.

Think of one very wonderful thing in your life. This can be an event or moment that gave you great unconditional pleasure, like the birth of your child, or falling in love with your mate. It has to be pure pleasure without any negative attachments. Focus on this.

The thing that you were so worried about asking yourself, "What if _____happened instead?"

This will quickly move out of your brain because it will feel contradictory. It will feel opposite to what you have created. Even

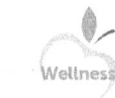

if it doesn't seem possible, just think as if you were creating a script or screenplay. Write it out the way you want it to go down. It's okay if it doesn't play out that way the first few times, you have only been practicing writing a new story for a short while in a positive way. How many times does it actually happen when you write the script in a negative way? Almost always! After a few times, the story will start to play out in a positive way that you have written, and you will feel the power of it.

If you still feel anxious and feel like the addiction has power over you, then go through the steps again.

I recommend reading, *Loving What Is* by Byron Katie and doing the work on old hurts and feelings. www.thework.com

Remember addictions are just a pattern interrupt. Commit to learning a new pattern interrupt that will heal your mind, body, and spirit!

Focus on what you want! Don't give into the fear.

If your life or health is not what you want it to be, then you and only you can change it! You can't keep doing the same thing you've always done and expect it to change.

Healing, wellness, and feeling fabulous is a journey. To be the fabulous you that you deserve to be, you must make true change in your life. You must start your journey. You must embrace change.

Two things hold us back from making change: "fear" and "lack of trust."
To embrace change, you may have to face your fears.

Fear can be protective, but what about when it keeps you from living the life you dream. What can you do about fear? How can you overcome it?

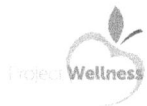

What are you afraid of?

Do this exercise! It will change your life.
Write down on a piece of paper all the things you are afraid of. List
them one by one. It can be a short list or long, but be honest. Then
burn the list. Place it in a tin can with a glass of water nearby and
watch the paper slowly burn. Take a deep breath and let the ritual
engulf you. Let it go. Let it all go! This is the first step. Then use
the tips that follow to live your life in love and trust—NOT FEAR!

Face your fear to become stronger.
If you lay in your bed and worry that a monster is in your closet,
you just create more anxiety for yourself. You secrete more
adrenaline and cortisol. Getting up and looking in the closet is the
best thing you can do. You know there is no monster there, and
it's just the fear that has built up in your mind. Well, you're not
nine years old and the monsters are bigger now than then, but the
principle still applies. If you are worried that your boss is mad at
you, go ask him. "Am I doing a good job?" "Is my job in
jeopardy?" "What could I do better?"
Regardless of his answer, you have faced your fear and you can
take action on improving your situation. This is only one example.
If you think someone is talking bad about you, just ask them and
find out why. Action is the best antidote to fear.

Don't take your fear so seriously. You might think to yourself that
what you thought was a fear before wasn't that much to be afraid
of at all. Everything is relative. And every triumph, problem, fear,
and experience becomes bigger or smaller depending on what you
compare it to.

But to gain a wider perspective of human experience and grow,
you really have to step up and face your fear. What if what you
want doesn't happen? What would your life look like? Just be
present with the thought. Don't try to push it under the rug.

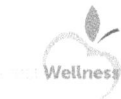

Get input from others. Make contact with the fear. Get in its face. Start working on your health and learning as much as you can about how to change your health and your situation.

99% of the things we worry about happening never happen, and 99% of the things that happen, that we should have worried about, we never thought of.

Fear is often based on false interpretation or miscommunication. As humans, it is our nature to look for patterns. The problem is just that we often find negative and not so helpful patterns in our lives based on just one or two experiences. Or by misjudging situations. Or through some silly miscommunication. Our brains make neuronal connections to past events. It is important not to judge past experience on future interactions. Every situation is different. We transfer a lot of fear and misgivings into future situations that we should really approach with a fresh perspective.

Don't cling to your illusion of safety. The only thing permanent is change and there is no "comfort zone."
One big reason why people don't face their fears is because they think they are safe where they are right now. But the truth is safety is only a sense; like fear, it is not real, only perceived. There is no safety out there, really. It is all uncertain and unknown.
Life happens, you may lose your job, your loved one, have to move, lose your home, or suffer unknown tragedy. You may get laid off. You will eventually die. Who knows what will happen? This perception of safety is not always a bad thing. It's protective. But there is also not that much point in clinging to an illusion of safety. So you need to find balance where you don't obsess about the uncertainty, but also recognize that it is there and live accordingly.
As you stop clinging to your safety, life also becomes a whole lot more exciting and interesting. You are no longer as confined by an illusion and realize that you set your limits for what you can do, and to a large extent, create your own freedom in the world. You

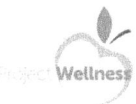

are no longer building walls to keep yourself safe as those walls wouldn't protect you anyway.

Be curious.

When you are stuck in fear, you are closed up. You tend to create division in your world and mind. You create barriers between you and other things/people.
How do you become more curious? One way is to remember how life has become more fun in the past, thanks to your curiosity, and to remember all the cool things it helped to discover and experience. And then to work at it. Curiosity is a habit. The more curious you are, the more curious you become. And over time it becomes more of a natural part of you.

Trust is another antidote to fear.

Most of our fears are based on how others perceive us.
The ego wants to divide your world. It wants to create barriers and loves to play the comparison game. The game where people are different compare to you, the game where you are better than someone and worse than someone else. All of that creates fear. Doing the opposite removes fear.

But one thought you may want to try for a day is that everyone you meet is your friend. To take this one step further, assume that every one you meet has something to teach you.

There is often an underlying frame of mind in interactions. Either it asks us how we are different to this person. Or how we are the same as this person. This creates warmth, an openness and curiosity within. There is no place to focus on fear or judgment anymore.

This is of course not easy, especially if you have held the first frame of mind for many years. But you can get insight into this by

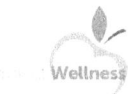

doing the rest of the things above. As you face your fears the barriers and separation you have built in your mind decreases. You come closer and feel more of a connection to other people.

With action, curiousness and understanding we come closer to each other. We gain a greater understanding of ourselves and others. And so it becomes easier to see them in you. And you in them.

Focus on Love
When you hold others and make physical contact a hormone called oxtocin is released in the brain. This is the love hormone that helps mothers to be affectionate and cuddle their babies. It is thought to be deficient in those with anxiety disorders and those with focus disorders or chronic pain, all physical manifestations of fear and lack of trust.

Here are ways to naturally boost your body's oxytocin production:

Hugs: Just embracing others, holding hands, or draping an arm around your significant other, child, or person you care for can produce an increase in oxytocin.

Make eye contact: When you interact with others oxytocin can be enhanced with mental embrace as well as physical contact.

Passion: Adults seeking an oxytocin surge should head for the bedroom. The hugging and touching during foreplay fires up the love chemical, and orgasm spikes the hormone level to two times the normal amount. This opens the door to a relaxed feeling and a greater opportunity to bond with your partner.

Get your hormones balanced: Interestingly, among premenopausal young women, oxytocin is naturally higher during ovulation because estrogen intensifies the love hormone. This may partially explain why women seem to be more prone to touch and other

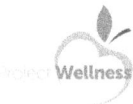

displays of affection during ovulation.

Get a pet: A loyal pet is there to make owners feel good. And because the release of oxytocin is triggered by touch, petting a dog or cat you love can also increase oxytocin levels.

2. Get healthy physically, exercise, take supplements that help with stress and focus on nutrition and learn to listen to what your body needs

The physical benefits of exercise are well known. While it removes toxins and build muscle, enhancing growth hormone, it also is important for mental fitness and reducing stress. It can improve alertness and concentration as well as overall cognitive function. Stress causes your brain to be bathed in cortisol, which can affect your ability to focus and your short term memory, so decreasing this response can actually improve memory as well.

Exercise produces endorphins, which are chemicals in the brain that act as natural painkillers. Many people are stressed with chronic pain. Even just 5 minutes a day can be enough to reduce stress and anxiety.

3. Recognize how you feel and honor it.

Denial is a powerfully protective reaction to stress. Short term it may provide some relief but until you honor your feelings and release them, they just stay stored up waiting for your brainstem to get triggered and stirred once again. All of our processing of situations as they happen is based on past experience. That's how we deal with the future by our observations of the past. It would be nice just to say, "stop doing that", but the way our brains process it is virtually impossible. This is why it is so important to not only honor what we are feeling but to go into an inquiry process of why we feel that way.

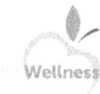

One way you can do this is to ask yourself, "When is the last time I felt that way?" Often times what you are dealing with in the present and all worked up about isn't even what you are really stressed about. It's something from your past that has you triggered and reactive.

One day I woke up and could not find my husband anywhere. No note. He didn't tell me he was going anywhere. It wasn't typical for him. He always tells me if he is leaving. We have only been married a few years, but in all that time, this was the first time that ever happened. As the minutes ticked by, I got more agitated. By the time he got home, I was really, really upset. He was confused. He had gone to the doughnut shop to get some treats for breakfast and surprise me. He thought I'd be sleeping for a while.

When I gave myself some time and just "sat with the feeling." I asked myself, "What are you really feeling and when was the last time you felt that way?"

What surfaced was when my dad died when I was nineteen. I wasn't home and didn't get to tell him goodbye. I never really dealt with that feeling. It was abandonment. It was anger, how could he do that, leave without saying goodbye? It was fear. It was alone. It was loss. All of that. It wasn't his fault of course that he died, but I was angry. How could he leave?

I had projected all those stored emotions to my poor husband who just went out for doughnuts. When I was able to really look at that I saw how silly it was that I was upset at my husband when I knew where the feelings really came from. So often we don't know where the feelings come from and we don't know why we feel as strongly as we do. We just do. And that's ok but if you don't inquire and explore, you don't grow and you stay stuck. And stuck can feel stressful. You feel dis-empowered. Disconnected and alone. It affects your relationships and then you really disconnect

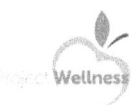

and feel alone. Then you feel guilt because you get reactive in your relationships and people don't put up with that for long. This is one of the ways that you can get addicted to another person. Setting yourself up in this reactive, needing forgiveness, guilt cycle. You realize that no one else would put up with this crap and you create this false sense of "needing" that other person because often they soothe you and help you to feel better in the moment.

We so often deny our feelings because it's just easier. We are taught as children not to cry, because it makes our parents uncomfortable when we are sad. Maybe because their parents were the same way. Generation to generation we are taught to suppress and disregard our sadness. Anger is just one emotion up from sadness and we are really taught to suppress that. Anger is just no okay to express in a civilized family.

I love any book by Marianne Williamson. One of the first books of hers that I read was during the breakup of a relationship. A friend of mine gave me the book and it really helped me through a very sad and difficult time. It's called *Return to Love* and one of the best things that I took away was to honor how I was feeling and that it was okay to cry. Tears release endorphins and oxytocin and rid the body of excess cortisol. I'm currently reading her book *Everyday Grace*, and she has such a great way of going through all the emotions that we feel and explaining that we just have to focus on honoring the feelings before they will fade or dissipate.

This is a great place where some "still" time, meditation, or prayer would come in helpful. Time to just reflect on how you are feeling and the last time you felt it. Bring it to the surface, honor it and then give it permission to leave. Once you give it permission to leave focus on how it might resurface in the future and then be ready to revisit it again should it appear. Don't fight it or think you should be bigger or more emotionally healthy than you are.

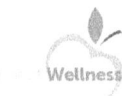

I have recently learned that the "shoulds" can be very destructive in your life. I didn't know why I was feeling the way I was. I was very anxious and uncomfortable in my life. I kept telling myself, "I should be happy." I have everything going for me and so much to be grateful for, but I wasn't happy. I didn't like my work life the way it was and kept telling myself, "I should be okay with this." Once my life coach identified that I was trapped in the "shoulds," I was able see that no matter how much you tell yourself you "should" feel this or that or be happy with a situation if you are not, then you are not, and no amount of "shoulds" can change that. This is the ultimate example of denial and is so destructive.

Now I just honor how I feel and have stopped telling myself, "I should…" It releases so much anxiety knowing that I can just be me. I also learned from my life coach that being uncomfortable means that you are getting ready to grow in a new direction. It's like being in the birth canal. It's so uncomfortable there. You can't stay. You have to keep going in the right direction. There is nothing you can do to stop it. The next step may be scary because it's the unknown but what you are feeling is normal. The anxiety is just the mind and the spirits way of acknowledging your transformation. When you stop fighting it you can embrace the experience and be ready for the new place in your life that you will find yourself in.

In this process you also have to learn to love yourself, which can be difficult for many people. Feeling inadequate seems to be in our DNA, but it is a learned response. When you can acknowledge that all of life is about growth and experience there are no failures. This is a myth. I love the book, *Conversations with God*, by Neal Donald Walsh.

It was so compelling as I read it that our ego develops myths so that we can protect our ego. One of the myths is that failure exists. When you think about your ego as the essence that separates you

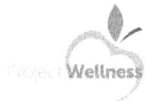

from all others, it must believe that failure exists, because we also believe the myth that scarcity exists. If scarcity exists then failure and success dictate who has abundance and who does not. One of the other myths is that we are separate from each other and separate from God and we are not. We are all connected at the soul. When we let go of these myths, we start to see that we are not alone, not failures, not loved or not good enough. All of this when it actually sinks down into the soul drives the ego away and protecting the selfish ego is what keeps us experiencing separateness so that we can now connectedness. All of life is about contrast and learning to know our true selves, not our ego as we have come to believe. We experience in the physical the up so that we can know down, happy so that we can know sad, scarcity so the we can know abundance… and on and on. It's all part of the plan and when I accepted these truths and learned to observe my ego as a protective part of me, it changed the way I view experiences.

I am in no way perfect and still experience anxiety from time to time, get caught up in my ego and feel separate and overwhelmed but I always come back to the "knowing" that it is just an experience. Which leads us to reality. What is reality? Reality is what we define it as. More about that coming up.

Spend some time thinking about what you want

Now that you have a deeper understanding of ego. You can begin to understand that ego is what drives us to "want things". Because one of the myths of the ego is that we have to do anything at all. The only thing we have to do is "be". There is enough love, enough of everything in every moment. But while we are splashing around in this thing called life and stroking our delicate egos, we are compelled to seek. We are compelled to grow and develop and the physical is our only frame of reference in which to do that, so we have drive to have things and create things. Let's face it. It's fun to build and experience what we have built. We feel much sense of accomplishment. It's what the ego does. So as

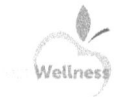
long as we are playing here, we might as well have things happen that we want.

There has been a great understanding of the "law of attraction" surfacing. The law of attraction states that what we think about most of the time is what we attract. We can think about good things and attract good things or focus on bad things and attract bad things. It is law. I have seen it in my life and everyone who is successful understands this law. Of course our definition of success is measured by the myth of scarcity and failure but focusing on good things will definitely manifest a more comfortable experience here for you.

As you spend time thinking about what you want, focus first on wanting to be happy and at peace. When friends of mine are fighting with their spouses or significant others, I usually ask them does it feel better to be right or be happy? The ego says, "right," but our true selves know the answer is "happy."

Once when my husband and I were having a little rough patch, a friend of mine told me this statement that has changed my life. "Seek to understand, not be understood." This is very hard for the ego because we want to be right and understood.

So many difficult times in my life with stressful disagreements the thing that kept me going was the thought, "I love this person and I want a peaceful relationship." I kept focusing on that.

Project Fun was born out of a need for stress reduction and these are the exercises for self-discovery, self-love, and goal setting.

"A life unexamined is a life not worth living." –Socrates

Seek to understand yourself and you'll understand the universe! Life is a *process*. A journey, not a destination. We are a work in progress. We never get it wrong and we never get it done. This

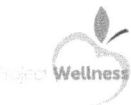

process will be the key to an extraordinary life. Emotion drives growth and progress. When you are uncomfortable with negative emotion it means you are preparing for the next phase of your life. Isn't it delicious? If you feel bad or comfortable, it's *awesome*. It means you are in the birth canal, or the cocoon ready to break free and become who you were always meant to be. Wanted to be. Maybe were afraid to be. Learn to embrace discomfort and see it as a guidance process to drive you where you want to go.

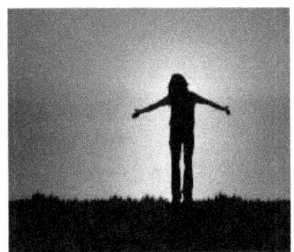

Don't make goals, make yourself **promises** to pursue self-discovery, life, being in the moment, and having fun!

4 steps to your process:

1. Self-discovery/awareness
2. Self Talk
3. Engage the magic of joy (Law of attraction) Gratitude Exercises
4. Question everything, be silly, have fun!

Here are some thoughts summarized that I found on my path that may be meaningful to me. These ideas reoccur over and over throughout the exercises. Print these out if you feel them to be meaningful to you or write your own and post them on your mirror, your refrigerator, etc and review them every morning and night.

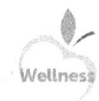

1. Thoughts become things
2. Words become beliefs
3. Beliefs become reality
4. Don't personalize anything
5. Close doors that need closing
6. Recognize the illusions of this physical life
   a. Separateness
   b. Failure
   c. Scarcity
   d. Judgment
7. Be thankful for every breath, every laugh, every day. Be thankful for unanswered prayers. Be Thankful for your eighty pennies.
8. Be the change (don't expect anyone else to change)
9. There is no such thing as right or wrong, just that which doesn't serve us or leads us away from who we truly are or our authentic selves.
10. There is no such thing as coincidence
11. You have all the answers, stop thinking you don't and stop telling yourself that
12. Everything that happens for you in this physical existence is for your growth and experience. You are responsible for EVERYTHING in your life. Stop making excuses and stop being a victim
13. Be still
14. Give it to God, he is bigger than any problem you have
15. Faith is all you need. Believe that everything happens for a reason and that everything always works out for you. Believe that it is all as it should be. Say "all is well" even when you don't feel it
16. There are only two emotions-love and fear- choose love
17. Fear is not bad, it is just an emotional indicator that we are off course. Embrace it
18. Visualize creatively every moment. Don't think about what you want but how it will feel in the having of it. That brings it quicker.

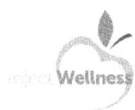

19. If you don't have anything good to say don't say anything at all, seriously!
20. Act as if
21. Exercise beautiful self talk and affirmations
22. If you want to be happy cause someone else to be happy
23. If you want abundance give something abundantly
24. If you want to be successful help make someone else successful
25. Focus on the way you want things not the way they appear to be
26. The universe only says "yes". If you say I want more money law of attraction says "yes you want more money" be aware of the belief underlying your request
27. Ego is necessary to keep you believing that you are in the illusion. True freedom is knowing that you are pure love energy here in this physical existence to know contrast
28. The only Zen that you find at the top of the mountain is the Zen you take with you
29. Use the word "should" to your advantage, think of all the reasons you should have abundance don't use should to talk yourself into doing things that others think you should, find your own path
30. Use reverse negativity in your words and questions, "why do people always say nice things to me?" "why is everything always working out for me?"
31. Embrace change. It is not only necessary but brings all the really cool stuff that you don't have right this minute, even the stuff that doesn't feel good in the process is always leading you on a path of experiencing contrast so that you know what you want
32. Acknowledge resistance and ask for help to see with new eyes the blessings that you are missing
33. Don't make goals, make yourself promises

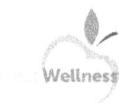

34. Speak ease into your life and always choose the path of least resistance
35. Don't judge ANYONE and certainly don't judge YOURSELF
36. Say "Hello Beautiful" to yourself every morning in the mirror
37. Always find ways to have fun. Be silly, trigger laughter all around. There is nothing more important than your happiness.
38. You choose how you feel in any moment. Stop being the victim and be happy.
39. Believe in infinite possibility
40. Reality is only what you define it to be. Watch the movie from the third row seat and enjoy. People pay money for the adrenaline rush you get from the delicious dangerousness of living a life well lived
41. Take risks. Lots of em!
42. You are limitless.
43. Everyone is right. Seek to understand not be understood. Everyone is right from where they stand and what they know. Seek to see it from their point of view. Think about the struggles that they experience and remember that it is more important to be happy than "right". Put yourself in other's shoes emotionally when you are confused at their behavior
44. See angry people as scared little kids
45. Embrace strangers, it could be an angel in disguise. Try to put yourself in their shoes if you feel judgment coming on
46. Think of problems as opportunities to grow
47. EXHALE
48. Understand your communication style
    -relator
    -socializer
    -thinker
    -director

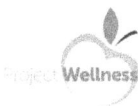
49. Know your love language
-service
-gifts
-affirmations
-affection
-quality time
50. Be curious.
51. Learn something new everyday

Want to know the secret to having the life of your dreams????
There is really only one thing that you need to implement in your
life.   Simple as it seems it is

## Lets have some fun, discover who you are and begin the exercises!!!

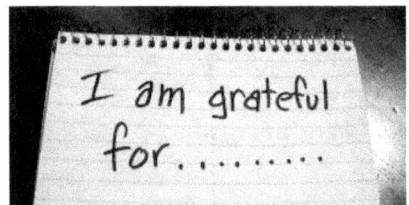

I am grateful for.........

"It is not happy people who are thankful but thankful people who are happy." -*unknown*

**Exercise 1:**  Think about this thought.  What if you woke up
tomorrow and all you had was what you are grateful for today?  If
you didn't feel grateful for your house or apartment?  Gone!  If
you weren't grateful for your spouse?  Gone.  If you weren't
grateful for your children?  Gone.  And the list goes on….
Wouldn't you wish you had been grateful?  When your teenager is
acting like "teenager" and you feel stressed about that, consider
this.  What if tomorrow they were gone.   Would all the things that
you are stressed about even matter?  All you would do is the
mourn the loss of that precious person in your life.  Right?  So the
biggest key in any moment is to focus on what you are grateful for

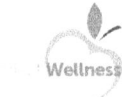
about the circumstance. Often we don't realize what we have until it's gone. We don't appreciate our mate and then they leave for someone else. We didn't even realize how much we appreciated them until they are gone. When your spouse goes out of town even for just a little while you realize all the things they do that you are grateful for when they are not there to do them.

Gratitude is the key to focusing on what is good your life so that you can attract more like it. This is the law of attraction. What you focus on (wanted or unwanted) is what you bring more of. If you focus on gratitude you cannot help but focus on the wanted in any situation.

Consider this, too. Have you ever known anyone that was not grateful? How negative is their energy? Do you like to be around that person? If your child is unappreciative of the toys they already have, do you feel like buying them more? If your spouse doesn't seem appreciative of the dinner you made and just complains, do you feel like ever making them dinner again?

God and the universe is the same way. God has put into place the universal law of attraction to give you everything you want. God only says yes. If you are unappreciative of what you have do you think that is lining you up to get more? And if God only says yes and you say "I don't like that I don't have any money, or stuff, or the ideal weight…etc." and you are merely complaining about what you don't have and not appreciating what you do have, do you think God is going to move the universe around to line up what you want next? Unlikely.

Being grateful is the key to getting more and keeping what you have that you love.

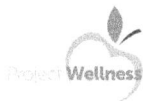
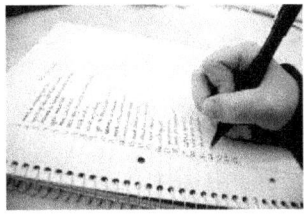

"Be yourself, everyone else is already taken." *–Oscar Wilde*

**Exercise 2:** Write your own truths and post them where you can read them each morning and night.

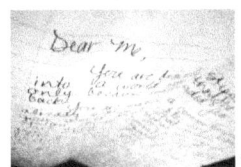
"If you make friends with yourself, you will never be alone." *– Maxwell Maltz*

**Exercise 3:** Write a letter to yourself thanking yourself for taking the time for this journey.

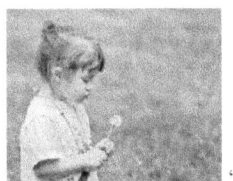
"We do not stop playing because we grow old, we grow old because we stop playing." *– Benjamin Franklin*

**Exercise 4:**

Childhood Photograph exercise:

Who am I?

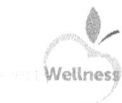
Wellness

Write about your childhood from your earliest memories to leaving home. Use different sensory descriptors, write the list in visual—what you saw, auditory—what you heard, physical—what you touched, olfactory—what you smelled. Use a different sheet of paper if you want to write more.

List all the *not* so good things about your childhood

_____
_____
_____
_____
_____
_____
_____

List all the really good things about your childhood

_____
_____
_____
_____
_____
_____
_____

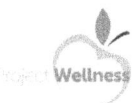 

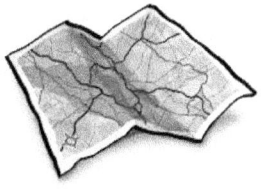

"No problem can be solved from the same level of consciousness that created it." *–Albert Einstein*

## Exercise 5:

Create your Life Map. A life map is a visual/text representation of what your life has looked like in the past, what it looks like now and the what the ideal life looks like that you wish to create. It's your "map" for the path to your own happiness. A life map involves visualizing (and then putting into writing) exactly what you want your life to look like in 7 specific areas: lifestyle & fun, career & work, money & finances, health & wellness, family & friends, love & romance and personal growth & spirituality. The process will take you through a linear process to create your own life map. Write out for each of the following categories what you have experienced in the past, what is currently happening and what you want to have happen in the next 1-3 years. The point of this exercise is to help you get clear on your future (don't think of the how's but the feelings of success, emotion, influence…)
**T** -thought, **I** -influence, **M** -manifestations, **E** -emotion

## Lifestyle and Fun:

Past

Present

Future

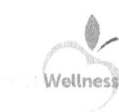

**Career and Work:**

Past

Present

Future

**Money and Finances:**

Past

Present

Future

**Health and Wellness:**

Past

Present

Future

**Family and Friends:**

Past

Present

Future

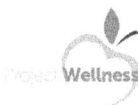

**Love and Romance:**

Past

Present

Future

**Personal Growth and Spirituality:**

Past

Present

Future

**Write your timeline of success, influence, and emotions:**

Begin with the end in mind-Stephen Covey.

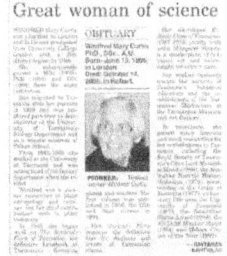

When you are born, you cry, and the world rejoices. When you die, you rejoice, and the world cries.
*-Buddha*

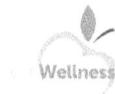
**Exercise 6:**

Write you obituary:
To help you map out your future… Do the following: write an obituary as a true account of your life to date. As an alternative, if you want to be more objective, as another exercise you can ask a friend or family member who knows you well to do one of you as well. When it's ready, look over your obituary and ask yourself questions such as the following:

If I died today, would I die happy?
Am I satisfied with the direction in which my life is headed?
Am I happy with the legacy that I'm creating?
What's missing from my life?
What do I need to do in order for my obituary to be "complete"?
Then, write a fantasy obituary in which you write down all of the things you wish you had done with your life. What does this exercise tell you? You're not dead yet, so get out there and start making any changes that you need to so that you can "live up" to your fantasy obituary.

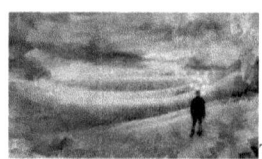
Thoughts become things. – *Mike Dooley*

"You yourself, as much as anybody in the entire universe, deserve your love and affection"
— *Gautama Buddha*

**Exercise 7:**
**Self Love**

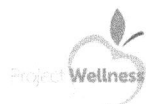

1.  Introduce yourself to yourself in the mirror. This exercise is like writing a Bio or resume.

Example: Tammy, I'd like you to meet Tammy. She is smart, funny, energetic, supportive and….. Really spend some time with this, talking to yourself.

> Forgive yourself for not taking better care of yourself
> Forgive yourself for forgetting who you really are
> Forgive yourself for abandoning your true identity

2.  Be easy on yourself, Lighten up. Commit to giving yourself a break. List all the ways you have been successful in relationships, work, etc. Think of your hardships not as proof of your unworthiness but evidence of your resiliency and resolve to not only survive, but thrive.
3.  Ask yourself the following questions:

"Who am I?"

"What do I need right now more than anything else?"

"What meaning can I draw from the toughest experience I ever had?"

"What feeling do I most want to have in my life? What do I want to be doing more of in my life? What do I want to be doing less of in my life?"

"What do I need to quit or cut out of my life?"

"What am I resisting, or attaching to?"

What are my gifts? What am I really good at? How can I share them with the world?

"How can I celebrate each day, or the moments of my life?"

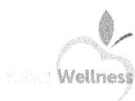

This exercise is designed to address the common emotions, situations and behaviors caused by a lack of self-love. Mirror work is the greatest gift you can give yourself. This powerful tool allows you to confront self-defeating behaviors and challenges you to choose love over all else. This life-changing decision will bring you numerous enriching benefits when you do the mirror work exercises and listen to medications, affirmations, and positive self-talk in this exercise.

"Know thyself." –*Socrates*

## Exercise 8:

Self Exploration:

10 Things that make me laugh

_____
_____
_____
_____
_____
_____
_____
_____
_____
_____

What person in your life makes you feel powerful?_____

Who makes you feel weak?(kryptonite)_____

My favorite color is:

_____

My favorite song is:

_____

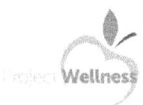

My favorite movie
is:_____
My favorite book is:

_____

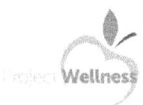

If I had a magic wand, these would be my 3 wishes:

_____
_____
_____

3 kind/nice things I have done lately:

_____
_____
_____

3 things I like most about my body:

_____
_____
_____

3 things I am really good at:

_____
_____
_____

If I could live anywhere in the world it would be

_____.

Why? _____

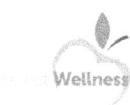
If I could close my eyes and appear anywhere it would be_____.

If I could be any animal I would be a:
_____

If I could change 3 things about myself:
_____
_____
_____

I'm scared of
_____
_____
_____
_____
_____
_____
_____
_____

My dream house would have:
_____
_____
_____

I would love it if my spouse would?
_____
_____
_____

If they made a movie about my life I would like
_____ to play me.

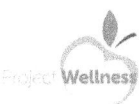

If they named an ice-cream after me it would be called:

_____

I deserve an award for:

_____
_____
_____

If I could be famous, I'd be famous
for_____

The best gift I ever got was

_____

The best gift I ever gave was

_____

Describe yourself as a
color_____

Family things that I like to do

_____
_____
_____

My hero is_____

The coolest person in my family tree is_____

If I could have any job in the world it would
be_____

If I worked in a hospital, I would be

_____

If I worked in a circus, I would be

_____

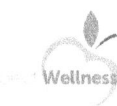

If I worked in a school, I would be

_____

Ten words that best describe me

_____
_____
_____
_____
_____
_____
_____
_____
_____
_____

**Need some help?**
Morning person
Night owl
Sporty
Artsy
Friendly
Loner
Clean freak
Tomboy
Princess/diva

If I could have one magical power it would
be_____

[]Invisible
[]Super hearing
[]See the future
[]Able to fly
[]Super strong
[]x-ray vision
[]other_____
Why?_____

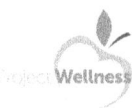

3 Things I never expected to happen in my life:

_____

_____

_____

What would make me feel really good about myself in the next 30 days?

_____

I always dreamed of doing_____

but _____told me I couldn't

because_____.

If I could do anything in the world without limitations it would be -

_____

I am judgmental of others who

_____

_____

_____

I don't like when other people judge me for

_____

_____

_____

These are behaviors I engage in when I feel happy

_____

_____

_____

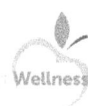
Wellness

These are behaviors I engage in when I don't feel happy or stressed

_____

_____

_____

These are the people that bring out the best in me

_____

_____

_____

These are the people that bring out the worst in me

_____

_____

_____

I feel in control when

_____

_____

_____

I feel out of control when

_____

_____

_____

My strengths are

_____

_____

_____

My weaknesses are

_____

_____

_____

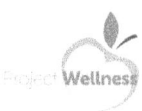

My happy ever after looks like

_____

_____

_____

(this is a trick question, we never get it wrong and we never get it done….HEE-HEE… gotcha)

These exercises will help you explore who you are and what you think about life.  Don't think too much about the process.  Just have fun with it.  The goal is to learn to know yourself a little better.  Knowing yourself can help you examine where you are in life and what your next steps should be.

**Exercise 9:**  Make a Vision Board

What is a vision board?

A vision board is a collage of images that represent your dreams. It could be words, pictures, places, material things all put together on a poster board or electronically made into a single image. The purpose of a vision board is to realize your future, and to activate your brain into moving in the direction of achieving what you desire and move from daydreaming to living your dreams.

What is the law of attraction?

The law of attraction is simple: whatever you project energetically or put your energy towards, whether that be positive or negative, you will attract. What you project is what you receive. A vision board is simply to help set our intentions for the way we want to live, and for our brains to pick up on that and make it happen. For example: If you say, "I will always be sick, I can't seem to get better. I feel terrible, and I'm stuck." Well guess what: You will be sick and you will be stuck. Your know theses people in your life. You brain hears whatever you say as truth. So your body isn't going to work towards healing if you believe you will always be sick; rather, it will work to fulfill that statement and make the thoughts match the reality.

The vision board therefore, is to help our brains recognize what it is we want to make true in our lives. It helps us unconsciously move towards our dreams in a very real and powerful way. If you are sick, then gravitate towards pictures that are of people healthy, active, smiling, and well. Repeat to yourself, "I am healthy, healed and full of energy"

How to create a vision board:

**Supplies Needed:**

- A large variety of Magazines in color (ask your friends, doctors office etc. for them) and/or images from your computer like Pinterest pages (print off)
- Scissors
- Poster Board, Foam Board or Cork Board
- Glue, Thumb Tacs, Cute Pins or Tape

**Process:**

Find images that convey your future and your dreams. Cut them out and/or print them out and arrange on a poster, foam or cork

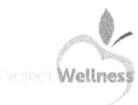

board. Attach them with glue or pins. Display in a prominent place that you will see everyday.

Each board is going to be as unique as the individual. However, there are a few tips and items you should considering incorporating into your board.

**Exercise 10:** Make a list of people who are where you want to be.
You don't have to reinvent the wheel. Study people who have been successful in the area you want to pursue. Study them, figure out how and why they are able to remain successful when everyone else is folding and then set up structures to emulate them. If you want to be creative, create a rigorous and formal plan. It's not the plan that is creative; it's the process that you go through that opens up so many possibilities.

**Exercise 11:** Start doing what you love, even without a specific plan.
A lot of people wait until they have an extensive business plan written down, along with angel investors wanting to throw cash at them -- and their ideas never see the light of day.

Do what you enjoy -- even if you haven't yet figured out how to monetize it. Test what it might be like to work in an area you're passionate about, build your network and ask for feedback that will help you develop and refine a plan.

It's a way to not only show the value you would bring, but you can also get testimonials that will help launch your vision when you're ready to make it official. Most

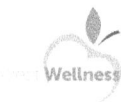

importantly, though, it'll shift you out of paralysis and fear and the joy of seeing the difference your contribution makes will fuel your creativity.

**Exercise 12:** Think about this thought. - Take a break from your usual thinking and take yourself on a "Creativity Date". I recommend you do this once a week. Make a date. Put it on your calendar and go see something new. This could be flea markets, museums, walk in a park, go to a business of something you wish you were doing and ask the owner if you could see how things work. While it might feel uncomfortable to step outside of your usual thinking mode, the mind sometimes needs a rest from such bottom-line thinking. Maybe schedule a class to help create a new hobby. Maybe you won't like it but maybe you will. Either way it will give you new contrast and experience. Maybe for you, it will be creative writing, painting, running or even gardening.

After you take a mental vacation indulging in something you're passionate about, come back to a journal and write down any ideas that come to mind.

"You'll be amazed at how refreshed your ideas are," he says. "Looking at beautiful things - art and nature - creates connections that we often neglect to notice. Notice them capture, them in writing and use them."

**Exercise 13:** Have FUN!

The Benefits of Play for Adults

Play is not just essential for kids; it can be an important source of relaxation and stimulation for adults as well. Playing with your romantic partner, co-workers, pets, friends, and children is a sure (and fun) way to fuel your imagination, creativity, problem-solving

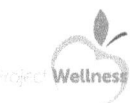

abilities, and improve your mental health. And actively playing with your kids will not only improve your own mood and wellbeing, it will make your kids smarter, better adjusted, and less stressed.

In our hectic, modern lives, many of us focus so heavily on work and family commitments that we never seem to have time for pure fun. Somewhere between childhood and adulthood, we've stopped playing. When we do carve out some leisure time, we're more likely to zone out in front of the TV or computer than engage in fun, rejuvenating play like we did as children. But just because we're adults, that doesn't mean we have to take ourselves so seriously and make life all about work. We all need to play.

Adult play is a time to forget about work and commitments, and to be social in an unstructured, creative way. The focus of play is on the actual experience, not on accomplishing any goal. There doesn't need to be any point to the activity beyond having fun and enjoying yourself. Play could be simply goofing off with friends, sharing jokes with a coworker, throwing a Frisbee on the beach, dressing up at Halloween with your kids, building a snowman in the yard, playing fetch with a dog, a game of charades at a party, or going for a bike ride with your spouse with no destination in mind. By giving yourself permission to play with the joyful abandon of childhood, you can reap the myriad of health benefits throughout life.

While play is crucial for a child's development, it is also beneficial for people of all ages. Play can add joy to life, relieve stress, supercharge learning, and connect you to others and the world around you. Play can also make work more productive and pleasurable.

Play can:

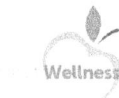
- **Relieve stress.** Play is fun and can trigger the release of endorphins, the body's natural feel-good chemicals. Endorphins promote an overall sense of wellbeing and can even temporarily relieve pain.
- **Improve brain function.** Playing chess, completing puzzles, or pursuing other fun activities that challenge the brain can help prevent memory problems and improve brain function. The social interaction of playing with family and friends can also help ward off stress and depression.
- **Stimulate the mind and boost creativity.** Young children often learn best when they are playing—and that principle applies to adults, as well. You'll learn a new task better when it's fun and you're in a relaxed and playful mood. Play can also stimulate your imagination, helping you adapt and problem solve.
- **Improve relationships and your connection to others.** Sharing laughter and fun can foster empathy, compassion, trust, and intimacy with others. Play doesn't have to be a specific activity; it can also be a state of mind. Developing a playful nature can help you loosen up in stressful situations, break the ice with strangers, make new friends, and form new business relationships.
- **Keep you feeling young and energetic.** In the words of George Bernard Shaw, "We don't stop playing because we grow old; we grow old because we stop playing." Playing can boost your energy and vitality and even improve your resistance to disease, helping you feel your best.

- **Play can heal emotional wounds.** As adults, when you play together, you are engaging in exactly the same patterns of behavior that positively shapes the brains of children. These same playful behaviors that predict emotional health in children can also lead to positive changes in adults. If an emotionally insecure individual plays with a secure partner,

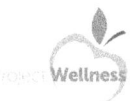 

for example, it can help replace negative beliefs and behaviors with positive assumptions and actions.

Many dot-com companies have long recognized the link between productivity and a fun work environment. Some encourage play and creativity by offering art or yoga classes, throwing regular parties, providing games such as Foosball or ping pong, or encouraging recess-like breaks during the workday for employees to play and let off steam. These companies know that more play at work results in more productivity, higher job satisfaction, greater workplace morale, and a decrease in staff turnover and absenteeism.

If you're fortunate enough to work for such a company, embrace the culture; if your company lacks the play ethic, you can still inject your own sense of play into breaks and lunch hours. Keep a camera or sketchpad on hand and take creative breaks where you can. Joke with coworkers during coffee breaks, relieve stress at lunch by shooting hoops, playing cards, or completing word puzzles together. It can strengthen the bond you have with your coworkers as well as help improve your job performance. For people with mundane jobs, maintaining a sense of play can make a real difference to the workday by helping to relieve monotony.

Success at work doesn't depend on the amount of time you work; it depends upon the quality of your work. And the quality of your work is highly dependent on your wellbeing.

**Playing at work:**

- keeps you functional when under stress
- refreshes your mind and body
- encourages teamwork
- helps you see problems in new ways
- triggers creativity and innovation
- increases energy and prevents burnout

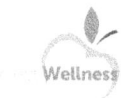
How To Put Fun Into Every Day

**1. Be where you are**.

Kids are really good at enjoying the moment. Adults are addicted
to thinking about all the things we have to do tonight, tomorrow,
next week. Where you are is where the fun is. Nowhere else.

**2. Get out of your comfort zone**.

Toddlers take risks all day long. As we mature, we tend to stay in
our safe place. Your day will be so much more exciting if you
gather the guts to wear hot pink pants.

**3. Smile 27 times more than you do**.

Children smile 400 times a day and adults, only 15. Smiling is the
catalyst to having fun.

**4. Notice nature**.

Every child is in awe of ants, birds, and dandelions. At some point,
we become creatures of the concrete jungle. Allow yourself to
be enamored by Mother Nature.

**5. Climb things**.

As soon as they discover their legs, kids start climbing everything.
There is something about being above ground level that is

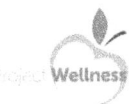

somewhat thrilling. Climb a rock. Climb a tree. You'll feel like the master of the universe.

**6. Embrace your "flaws."**

Being self-conscious is stifling.

**7. Use your imagination.**

A child can get lost in her make-believe world for hours. Imagine riding an elephant in Thailand. Or running a marathon on the Great Wall of China. You'll have so much fun pretending that you might want to make it a reality, which leads to more fun than you can imagine.

**8. Be unpredictable.**

There is no knowing what a kid will get up to next. Step out of your ordinary routine and you'll be surprised at how liberated you'll feel.

**9. Hand out high-fives.**

For no reason at all, kids hand out high-fives like they just won gold at the Olympics. Next time you hear some good news, give somebody a high-five. It feels good to get pumped about the little things.

**10. Slow down.**

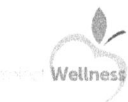
Children know how to take their sweet time. Allow yourself enough time to enjoy living. Rushing sucks all the fun out of the day.

**11. Create**.

Paint, draw, build, write. Kids clearly enjoy those activities. Fun is being in your creative element.

**12. Get dirty**.

Kids aren't afraid to experience life hands on. Get right in there. Make sandcastles. Turn up a log.

**13. Break the rules**.

Fun doesn't follow all the rules. Neither do kids. If it doesn't hurt, go for it! Leave those pretty Christmas lights up year-round.

How can you add more fun to your day?

**14. Break the rules**.

Buy some dollar pranks, learn some magic tricks, learn to make balloon animals.

**15. Skip**

You can't not have fun or laugh when you are skipping.

**16. Coloring!**

232

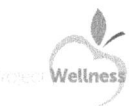

Buy some coloring books and crayons. Too fun.

## 17. Racing!

Perhaps the simplest idea of the bunch, racing is a great way to encourage healthy competition while getting some exercise. You can race your co-workers on the way to the bathroom to get to your favorite stall first. You can race to the elevator and quickly close the door on the person you were walking with. You can always race your dog while on a walk.

**Tips to engage in adult play:**

1. Don't overanalyze what you like to do or when you would like to do it.

2. Don't worry about what the neighbors will think. If you hear, "What's gotten into you?" You're on the right track.

3. Embrace simplicity.

4. Look at your old photos for a reminder. Which stand out more: the candid shots or the posed all dressed-up ones?

5. Create a special fun activity for those dreaded Monday mornings like a power breakfast with a friend or colleague.

6. Check your newspaper for free fun like concerts, films and fairs.

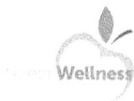 

If you don't know what to do for fun, ask yourself, "What did I do for fun when I was 10 years old?" You'd probably enjoy that activity now. Exploring the woods, playing with your dog, making things with your hands, riding your bike, baking, dancing around the room singing...think of ways to adapt this childhood fun to your life as an adult.

When I started to think about fun, though, I realized the importance of silliness; a happy atmosphere isn't created merely by the absence of nagging and yelling. I made a resolution to "make time to be silly." Studies show that in a phenomenon called "emotional contagion," we unconsciously catch emotions from other people, whether good moods or bad moods. Taking the time to be silly means that we're infecting one another with good cheer.

So in closing, remember that all the pillars are essential to health and wellbeing. Have fun with all of this and make it your lifestyle. A new beginning!

A year from now, will you wish you would have started now?

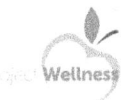

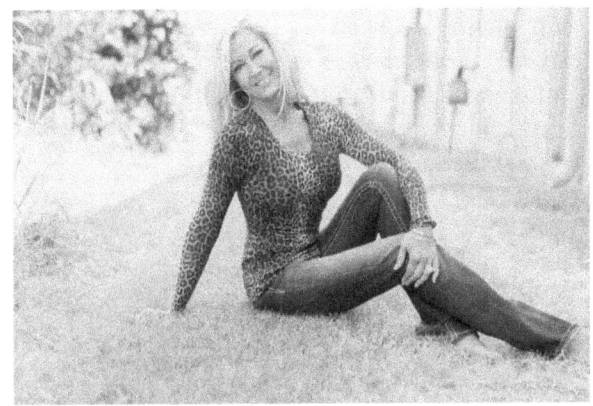

## ABOUT THE AUTHOR

Dr. Tammy has spent many years cultivating a culture of accountability in patients. She has motivated and mentored many in the ways of improving their own health one healthy decision at a time. Born and raised in a small town in Arkansas, she pursued her training all throughout the U.S. and is grounded and in tune with the simple to the sophisticated when it comes to educating her patients. Her extensive work and educational background lends to her non-traditional physician approach. She went beyond attaining a bachelor's degree in biology to pursing her master's degree in public health. While doing this, she began teaching and discovered a passion for educating as a means to spawn greatness and discovery in others. She then attended 4 years of medical school at Kansas City University of Medicine and Biosciences, plus an additional year at Truman Medical Center as a Pathology fellow, teaching and learning about the basics of human processes. Her goal was to integrate all these experiences, so she could be the best family physician and health educator/mentor possible. She did her residency in Tallahassee, Florida. She is currently a board-certified family practice physician licensed to practice in the state of Arkansas.

She has done award-winning research in multiple areas including education, cancer, and biologic hormone processes. She has focused additional emphasis on programs promoting wellness and preventive care. She offers her patients a unique approach to medicine by bringing an extensive education, a desire to help others, and a genuine desire to make the medical experience a positive one for all patients. She empowers patients to take charge of their own wellbeing and health through the balance of hormones, stress reduction, detox, supplements, and fitness. Oh, and she brings a BIG SMILE! Those who know her

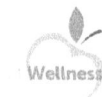

will confirm she loves enlightening, educating, and empowering others to pursue healthy lifestyles. She has spent the past few years transforming into everything she recommends. She definitely practices what she preaches!

www.ingramcontent.com/pod-product-compliance
Lightning Source LLC
Chambersburg PA
CBHW080244290526
45790CB00005B/1697